Manual on

HYSTEROSCOPY

Manual on HYSTEROSCOPY

Series Editors

Nandita Palshetkar
MD FCPS FICOG FRCOG (UK)
Professor Emeritus
Department of Obstetrics and Gynecology
DY Patil School of Medicine
Navi Mumbai, Maharashtra, India
Founder and Medical Director of the
Famous Bloom IVF Group

Hrishikesh D Pai
MD FRCOG (UK-HON) FCPS FICOG MSc (USA)
Trustee, FIGO, Asia Oceania (2023–25)
Professor, DY Patil University
Navi Mumbai, Maharashtra, India
Immediate Past President FOGSI (2022–23)
Founder and Medical Director
Bloom IVF Group, Mumbai

Niranjan Chavan
MD FICOG FCPS DGO DFP MICOG DICOG Diploma in Endoscopy (USA)
Professor and Unit Chief
Department of Obstetrics and Gynecology
Lokmanya Tilak Medical College and General Hospital
Mumbai, Maharashtra, India

Editors

Manoj Chellani
MBBS DGO DRM CIMP FICOG FIMS FMAS
Chairperson
Medical Disorders in
Pregnancy Committe, FOGSI
Director, Aayush Test Tube Baby Center
Raipur, Chhattisgarh, India

Nilesh Balkawade
MBBS MS DNB (Obs & Gyne) MNAMS
Fellowship in Reproductive Medicine
Diploma in Gyne Endoscopy (Kiel, Germany)
Chairperson, FOGSI Quiz Committee
2nd Joint Secretary AMOGS, Treasurer, MSR
Regional Medical Head, Oasis Fertility
Pune, Maharashtra, India

Rajendra Sankpal
MD DNBE FCPS DGO DFP European Diploma Gynec Endoscopy
Gynecological Endoscopic Surgeon
Dr Sankpal's Advanced Gynaecological Endoscopy Centre (SAGE Hospital), Mumbai
President Elect Mumbai Obstetric and Gynecological Society
Past President IAGE
Honorary Member ESGE

Co-Editors

Alka Kriplani, S Shantha Kumari, Krishnakumar, Siddhesh Iyer, Rohan Krishnakumar, Unnati Mamtora

JAYPEE BROTHERS MEDICAL PUBLISHERS
The Health Sciences Publisher
New Delhi | London

Message from Series Editors

Dear AICOG 2025 delegates,

It is a matter of great pride that the landmark AICOG 2025 is being held in the city of Mumbai, Maharashtra, India. The Organizing Committee and the hosts Mumbai Obstetric and Gynaecological Society have left no stone unturned in their quest to make this a historic event by aiming to have a scientific program of the highest caliber, punctuated by fantastic keynotes and orations, graced by the best international faculty in the field of Obstetrics, Gynecology and its subspecialities along with a cultural treat every evening to cater to the audience which hails from far-flung corners of India and the globe.

On this occasion, the academic stalwarts and senior FOGSIans have burned the midnight oil at both ends to contribute and create a set of AICOG 2025 Workshop Manuals that aim to amalgamate the most recent scientific advancements and evidence-based best practices in a nutshell for the delegates to take home and implement in their practices when they have returned from this magnificent event.

We acknowledge the efforts of all the editors, co-editors, authors, co-authors, co-contributors and junior authors who have sometimes worked at short notice to submit excellent chapters and articles included in the final publication. We also wish to take this opportunity to thank Shri Jitendar P Vij (Group Chairman) and Mr Ankit Vij (Managing Director) of M/s Jaypee Brothers Medical Publishers (P) Ltd, New Delhi, India, in publishing the book and their associates, particularly Ms Chetna Malhotra (Senior Director—Professional Publishing, Marketing, and Business Development), Ms Kritika Dua (Senior Commissiong Editor), and Mr Priyansh Saxena (Development Editor), who have been prompt, efficient, and most helpful.

We hope that the delegates and the attendees will enjoy reading this publication and the scientific data included therein will help to shape your knowledge, attitudes and practices and ultimately benefit the women of our country, whom we all serve.

Nandita Palshetkar
Organizing Chairperson, AICOG Mumbai, 2025

Hrishikesh D Pai
Chairperson, Scientific Committee, AICOG Mumbai, 2025

Niranjan Chavan
Organizing Secretary, AICOG Mumbai, 2025

FOGSI

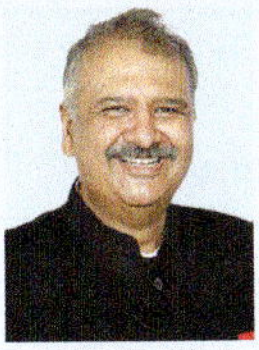

Jaydeep Tank
President 2024–2025

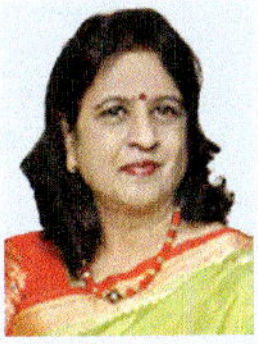

Madhuri Patel
Secretary General

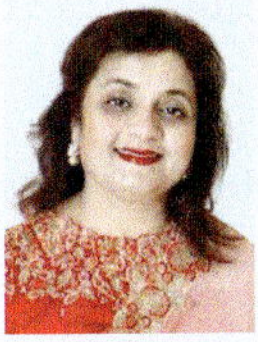

Sunita Tandulwadkar
President 2025–2026

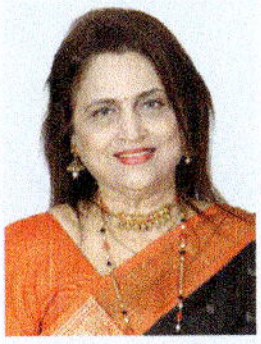

Suvarna Khadilkar
Deputy Secretary General

AICOG 2025 Core Committee

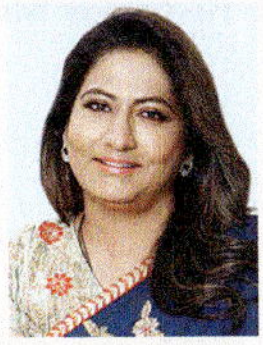

Nandita Palshetkar
Organizing Chairperson

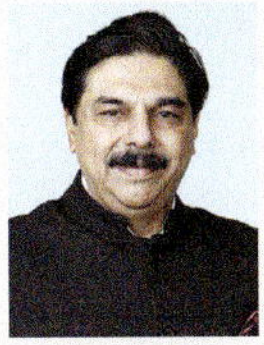

Hrishikesh D Pai
Chairperson, Scientific Committee

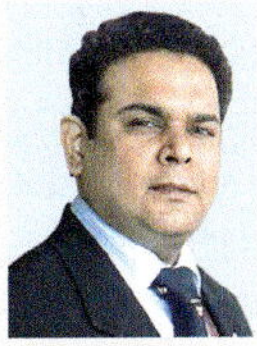

Niranjan Chavan
Organizing Secretary

Editors

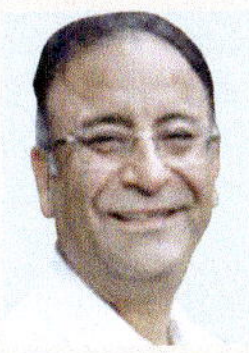

Manoj Chellani

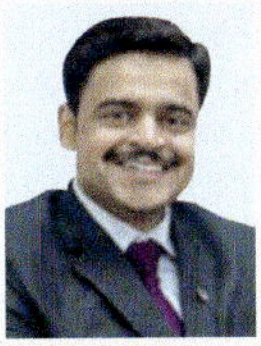

Nilesh Balkawade

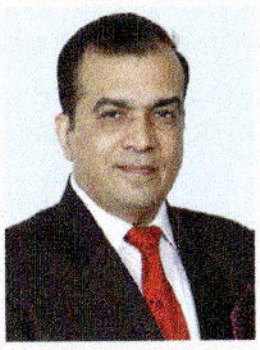

Rajendra Sankpal

Vice Chairpersons

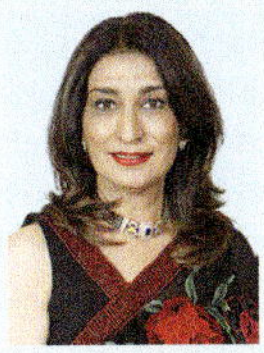

Rishma Dhillon Pai

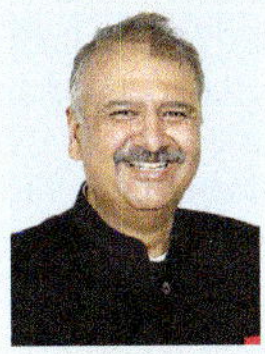

Jaydeep Tank

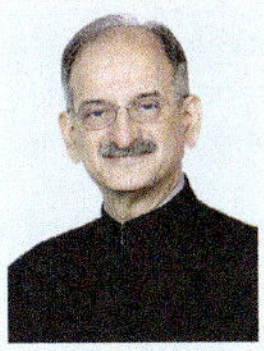

Nozer Sheriar

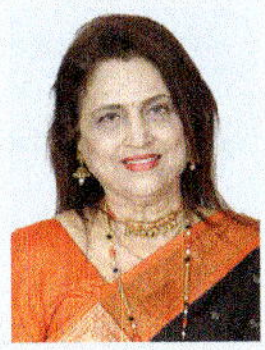

Suvarna Khadilkar

AICOG 2025 Publication Committee

Pratik Tambe	**Rohan Palshetkar**
Pradnya Supe	**Manan Boob**

JAYPEE **Jaypee Brothers Medical Publishers (P) Ltd**

Headquarters
EMCA House, 23/23-B
Ansari Road, Daryaganj
New Delhi 110 002, India
Landline: +91-11-23272143, +91-11-23272703
+91-11-23282021, +91-11-23245672
e-mail: jaypee@jaypeebrothers.com

Corporate Office
4838/24, Ansari Road, Daryaganj
New Delhi 110 002, India
Phone: +91-11-43574357
Fax: +91-11-43574314
e-mail: jaypee@jaypeebrothers.com

Overseas Office
JP Medical Ltd.
83, Victoria Street, London
SW1H 0HW (UK)
Phone: +44-20 3170 8910
e-mail: info@jpmedpub.com

EU GPSR Authorised Representative
Logos Europe, 9 rue Nicolas Poussin 17000,
La Rochelle, France
Phone: +33 (0) 6 67 93 73 78
e-mail: contact@logoseurope.eu

Website: www.jaypeebrothers.com
Website: www.jaypeedigital.com

Manual on Hysteroscopy

First Edition: **2025**

ISBN: 978-93-6616-762-6

Printed in India

Contributors

Amogh Chimote
MBBS MD FMAS BMAS
Medical Director
Vaunshdhara Fertility Centre, Nagpur
Assistant Professor
Shalinitai Meghe Hospital and
Research Center
Nagpur, Maharashtra, India

Anupama Bhute
MBBS DGO DNB PhD DIPMAS
FMAS FICOG Masters in Reproductive
Medicine and IVF (UK)
Assistant Professor
Datta Meghe Medical College
Nagpur, Maharashtra, India

Chaitanya Shembekar
MD FICOG FICMCH Diploma in Pelviscopy
Chairman and Managing Director
Omega Hospital, Shembekar
Hospitals Pvt. Ltd.
Nagpur, Maharashtra, India

Chiranjeev Shetty MBBS
Junior Resident
Department of Obstetrics and
Gynecology
DY Patil School of Medicine
Navi Mumbai, Maharashtra, India

Deepika Dewani
MBBS MD DNB (Obs & Gyne)
FMAS DMAS (Kiel, Germany)
Associate Professor
Department of Obstetrics and
Gynecology
JNMC DMIHER
Wardha, Maharashtra, India
President, DSOGS 2024

Deepti Gupta
MBBS MS DNB FICOG
Associate Professor
Department of Obstetrics and Gynecology
NSCB MCH, Jabalpur
Consultant and Unit Head
Ankur Fertility Clinic
Jabalpur, Madhya Pradesh, India
Secretary AMPOGS, NCE JOGI,
West Zone Coordinator, FOGSI Quiz
Committee

Gaetano Riemma
MD PhD
Candidate and Gynecologist
Obstetrics and Gynecology Unit
Department of Woman, Child and
General and Specialized Surgery
University of Campania
"Luigi Vanvitelli"
Naples, Italy

Manoj Chellani
MBBS DGO DRM CIMP FICOG FIMS FMAS
Chairperson
Medical Disorders in Pregnancy
Committe, FOGSI
Director, Aayush Test Tube
Baby Center
Raipur, Chhattisgarh, India

Mayuri More
MBBS MS (Obs & Gyne) FRM (ICOG)
DRM (Germany)
Consultant
DY Patil Fertility Centre (Bloom IVF),
Navi Mumbai
Assistant Professor
DY Patil School of Medicine
Navi Mumbai, Maharashtra, India

Megha Karnik
MBBS MS DNB (Obs & Gyne) Fellowship in Gyne Endoscopy
Diploma in ART, University of Kiel, Germany
Assistant Professor
Department of Obstetrics and Gynecology
JNMC, DMIHER (DU)
Wardha, Maharashtra, India
Secretary, DSOGS

Narendra Malhotra
MBBS MD FICOG FICMCH
FRCOG FICS FMAS AFIAP
Managing Director
Global Rainbow Healthcare
Ujala Cygnus Rainbow Hospital
Agra, Uttar Pradesh, India

Neema Acharya
DNB PHD FICOG MNAMS DGO DFP
Professor and Head
Department of Obstetrics and Gynecology
JNMC DMIHER
Wardha, Maharashtra, India

Neharika Malhotra
MBBS MD (Obs & Gyne) FICMCH FMAS
Infertility Consultant
Department of Gynecology
Rainbow IVF
Agra, Uttar Pradesh, India

Nilesh Balkawade
MBBS MS DNB (Obs & Gyne) MNAMS
Fellowship in Reproductive Medicine
Diploma in Gyne Endoscopy (Kiel, Germany)
Chairperson, FOGSI Quiz Committee,
2nd Joint Secretary AMOGS
Treasurer, MSR
Regional Medical Head, Oasis Fertility
Pune, Maharashtra, India

Rohan Palshetkar
MS (Obs & Gyne) FRM BDRME ADRME
Professor
DY Patil Medical College
Unit Head of DY Patil Bloom IVF and Opera House Bloom IVF
Chairperson of the FOGSI Young Talent Promotion Committee

Salvatore Giovanni Vitale
MS PhD in Medical and Surgical Biotechnologies
Assistant Professor
Division of Gynecology and Obstetrics
Department of Surgical Sciences
University of Cagliari
Cagliari, Italy

Sharayu Bhagat
MBBS MS (Obs & Gyne)
Junior Consultant
Oasis Fertility
Pune, Maharashtra, India

Stefania Saponara
MS PhD in Medical and Surgical Biotechnologies
Resident
Division of Gynecology and Obstetrics
Department of Surgical Sciences
University of Cagliari
Cagliari, Italy

Tanvir Singh
MBBS MS (Obs & Gyne)
Consultant
Tanvir Hospital
Hyderabad, Telangana, India

Preface

Hysteroscopy has evolved as a cornerstone in modern gynecology, transforming the way we diagnose and treat a wide variety of uterine conditions. This minimally invasive procedure offers unparalleled insight into the female reproductive system, enabling gynecologists to manage many complex cases with greater precision, safety, and efficacy. The purpose of this book is to provide a comprehensive guide to hysteroscopy, drawing on the latest advancements, techniques, and clinical insights to support both novice and experienced practitioners.

In this book, we delve deeply into the fundamentals of hysteroscopy, beginning with the history and evolution of the technique, before progressing to an in-depth exploration of the tools, procedures, and innovations that define contemporary practice. The chapters are organized to address the key aspects of hysteroscopy, from the initial patient evaluation and preparation, to diagnostic and operative procedures, complications, and post-operative care.

Throughout, we emphasize a multidisciplinary approach, recognizing that hysteroscopy is not only a valuable diagnostic tool but also an important therapeutic modality. The insights provided here are intended to help clinicians not only improve their technical skills but also enhance their decision-making and patient care.

This book aims to bridge the gap between theory and practice. Each chapter offers step-by-step instructions, supported by high-quality images and illustrations, to ensure clarity and ease of understanding.

As practitioners in the field of gynecology, we are continuously presented with new challenges and opportunities for advancing patient care. This book aims to equip gynecologists with the knowledge, tools, and confidence to navigate these challenges with expertise. Whether you are new to hysteroscopy or looking to refine your skills, this resource will provide invaluable guidance on enhancing your practice.

I hope this book serves as both a practical manual and a source of inspiration for all gynecologists dedicated to improving women's health through the power of hysteroscopy.

Series Editors: Nandita Palshetkar, Hrishikesh D Pai, Niranjan Chavan
Editors: Manoj Chellani, Nilesh Balkawade, Rajendra Sankpal
Co-Editors: Alka Kriplani, S Shantha Kumari, Krishnakumar, Siddhesh Iyer, Rohan Krishnakumar, Unnati Mamtora

Contents

1

CHAPTER

Instrumentation in Hysteroscopy

Deepika Dewani

Hysteroscopy is a procedure which is both diagnostic and operative. The various operative procedures which are done by hysteroscopic approach include excision of uterine polyp, submucous myoma excision, resection of uterine septum, tubal sterilization.[1]

INTRODUCTION TO HYSTEROSCOPIC INSTRUMENTATION

The success and safety of hysteroscopy heavily depend on the appropriate selection and use of specialized instruments.[2]

KEY COMPONENTS[3]

1. Sheaths
2. Endovision system (Telescope, Camera, Light source)
3. Electrosurgical instruments, cold instruments

SHEATHS

The telescope is fitted with a sheath so as to enable the infusion of distension media into the uterine cavity for panoramic viewing.

Types of Hysteroscopic Sheaths

Diagnostic

The diameter of the diagnostic sheath is 4–5 mm with approx. 1 mm clearance between the sheath and the telescope. A 5-mm instrument is usually easily passed through the endocervical canal and beyond the internal os with doing any cervical dilatation **(Fig. 1)**.

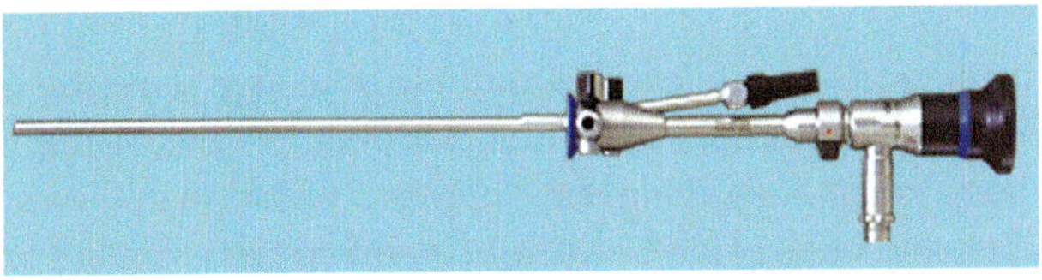

Fig. 1: A 3-mm telescope system.

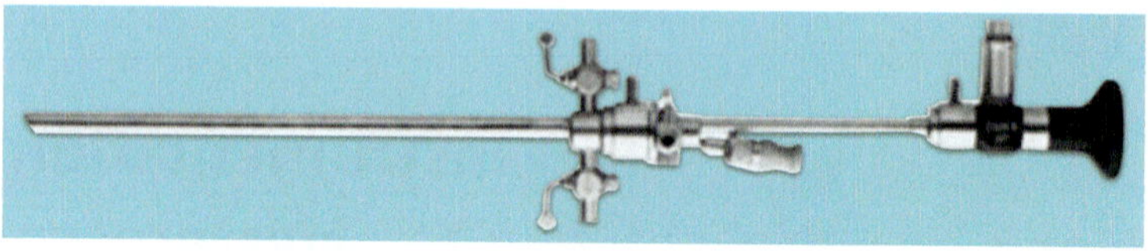

Fig. 2: Assembled operative hysteroscope.

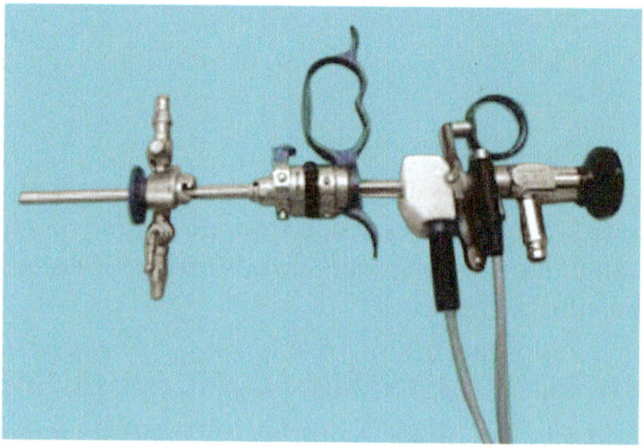

Fig. 3: Assembled resectoscope (coupled to a 30° telescope).

Operative

The diameter of operative sheaths is from 7 to 10 mm and there is space for insertion of operating device and inflow for distension medium. There is a rubber gasket which is used to seal the operating channel thereby preventing the leak of distension media. The newly developed sheath has a resectoscope along with the operative hysteroscope **(Fig. 2)**.

Resectoscope:

- It is an electrosurgical endoscope.
- It has an outer and inner sheath and allows usage of both monopolar and bipolar electrode devices.
- It comes with a 30° telescope.
- Diameter of an outer sheath is 8 mm or more hence, dilatation of cervix is required **(Fig. 3)**.

PARTS OF ENDOVISION SYSTEM

Telescope

There are three parts to a telescope, namely objective lens, the barrel and the eye piece. The sharpest, clearest image is obtained by a 4-mm telescope, and it also has a small outer diameter. There is a variation in viewing angle of telescopes. The telescope could be a 0° and therefore has a straight on view or a 30° telescope which has a fore oblique view and is commonly used **(Fig. 4)**.[4]

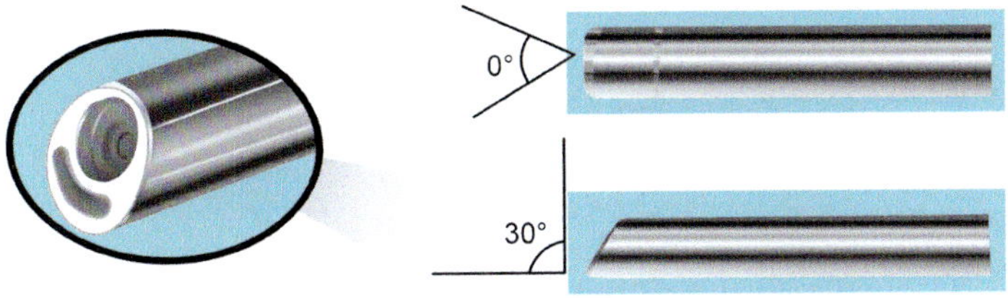

Fig. 4: 0° or 30° telescope.

Camera

There are various camera systems available which vary in sensitivity (Lux), resolution, the quality of the reproduction/video images. Now with improvisation in the technology, there is availability of high-definition cameras which have high resolution as well as natural color reproduction.[5]

Light Source

Parts of Light Source

Lamp/bulb: For light emission

Condensing lens: For vision

Fan: For reducing the temperature of light

Types of Light Source

- *Halogen:* It gives yellow colored light, produces more heat.
- *Xenon:* It consists of quartz glass. It gives better tissue differentiation.
- *LED:* It provides cold light, light intensity equivalent to xenon, lower power consumption, advanced technology, average life >50000 hours.

Light Cable

Working principle: Total multiple internal reflections

Light cable: They are of two types:

1. *Fiberoptic cable **(Fig. 5)**:*
   Fiber size: 10–25 mm diameter
   - Made up of a bundle of optical fiber glass thread.
   - They are fragile with good quality transmission.
   - Maintenance is easier.
2. *Liquid crystal gel cable:*
   - Made up of liquid crystal or clear optical gel.
   - Transmits approx. 30% more light than optic cable.
   - They have more transmission of heat than fiber optic cable.

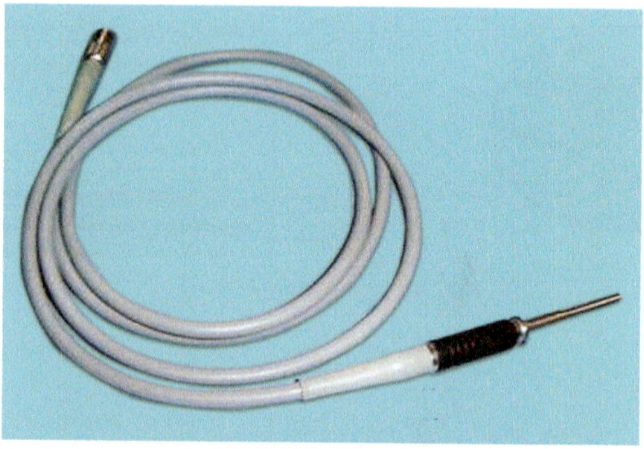

Fig. 5: Fiberoptic cable.

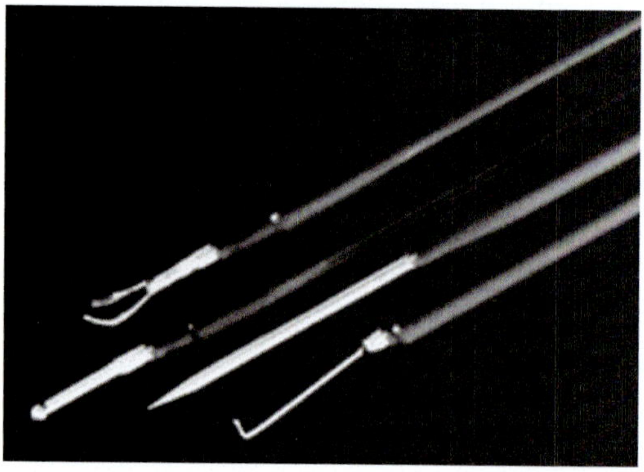

Fig. 6: *Electrodes (top to bottom):* Loop electrode, ball electrode, needle, and hook electrode.

ACCESSORY INSTRUMENTS

- *They are of two types:* Semirigid and flexible
- The semirigid instruments are small in size, hence fragile and prone to breakage, whereas flexible devices are less prone to breakage.
- They are with a diameter of 2–3 mm.
- *They include the following:* Electrosurgical electrodes, scissors, biopsy forceps, and grasping forceps **(Figs. 6 and 7)**.[6]

Hand Instruments

Figures 7A to C shows the hand instruments, e.g., biopsy/grasping forceps, pointed scissors, and tenaculum.

FLUID MANAGEMENT SYSTEMS/IRRIGATION SYSTEMS (FIG. 8)

- *Gravity fall of liquid*: The bag is suspended at a suitable height (90–100 cm from the patient's perineum is sufficient to obtain an irrigation pressure of approx. 70 mm Hg).

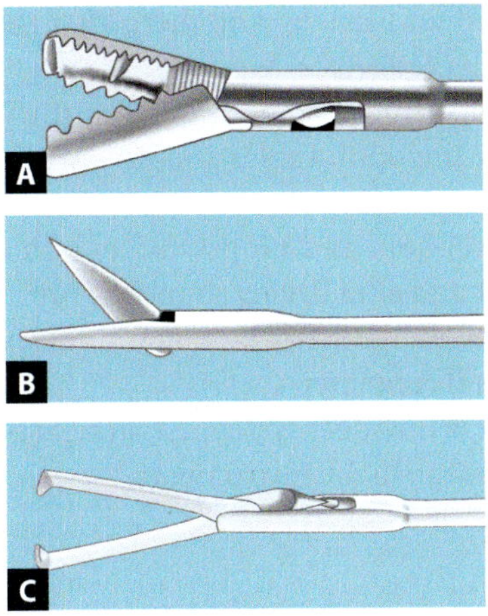

Figs. 7A to C: (A) Biopsy/grasping forceps; (B) Pointed scissors; (C) Tenaculum.

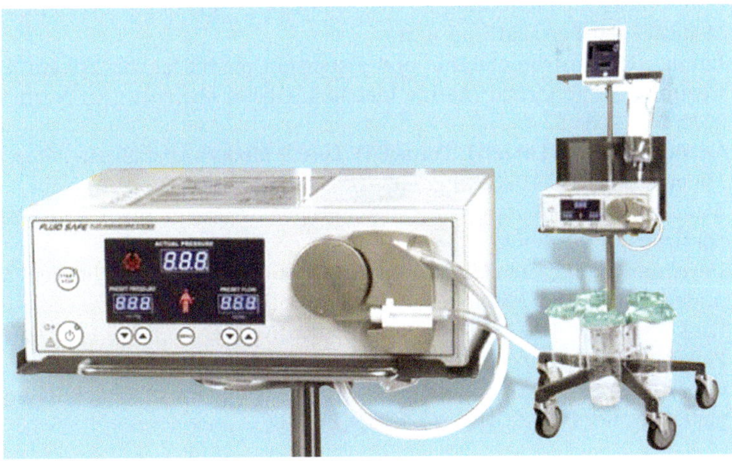

Fig. 8: Fluid management system.

- *Pressure cuff:* The pressure is obtained by inflating the pressure cuff and must be kept at around 80 mm Hg by an assistant.
- *Electronic suction and irrigation pump:* It has set values parameters like flow rate, irrigation pressure, suction pressure. This device enables controlling the flow rate as well as monitoring as well as adjustment of the preset volumetric difference between the in- and outflow irrigation liquid.[7]

MAINTENANCE AND STERILIZATION OF INSTRUMENTS

- Cleaning of telescopes and lenses should be done with utmost care.

- Warm water is used for washing and there after the endoscope must be cleaned with cotton pledgets.
- Special disinfectants should be used to clean the fiber optic cables and later while storage the optic cables should always be arranged in large loops.
- Instruments like scissors and biopsy forceps should be first cleaned, rinsed under water and after drying should be lubricated.
- Endoscopes when undergo sterilization by autoclaving should be placed in a perforated metal container.
- Ethylene oxide gas is the ideal system for sterilization as it works on low hence minimal damage to the instruments.[8]

REFERENCES

1. Mencanglia L, Cavalcanti L, Neto A, Alvarez AA. Manual of hysteroscopy—diagnostic, operative and office hysteroscopy. Tuttingen: Endo Press; 2013.
2. History and evolution of hysteroscopy. In: Shawki O, Deshmukh S, Pacheco LA (Eds). Mastering the techniques in hysteroscopy. New Delhi: Jaypee Brothers Medical Publishers; 2017. pp. 8-21.
3. Indman PD. Instrumentation and distension media for the hysteroscopic treatment of abnormal uterine bleeding. Obstet Gynecol Clin North Am. 2000;27(2):305-15.
4. Centini G, Troia L, Lazzeri L, Petraglia F, Luisi S. Modern operative hysteroscopy. Minerva Ginecol. 2016;68(2):126-32.
5. Blanc B, Marty R, Montgolfier R. Office and operative hysteroscopy. Paris: Werlag Springer; 2013. (e-Book).
6. Development of hysteroscopy from a dream to a reality and its linkage to the present and future. J Minim Inv Gynecol. 2007;14(4):407-18.
7. Rock JA, Jones III HW. Te Linde's Operative Gynecology, 11th edition. Philadelphia: Lippincott Williams & Wilkins; 2015.
8. Cohen S, Greenburg JA. Hysteroscopic morcellation for treating intrauterine pathology. Rev Obstet Gynaecol. 2011;4(2):73-80.

2

CHAPTER

Basics of Distension Media and Energy Sources Used during Hysteroscopy

Neema Acharya

Hysteroscopy is visualization of uterine cavity, and its structure by a telescope (hysteroscope). It is necessary that clinicians and surgeons practicing hysteroscopy are well verse with the basics of the equipment and instrumentation used during hysteroscopy. The following chapter deals with the basics of distension media and energy sources used during hysteroscopic surgery. The readers can go through the details of these topics and the related evidence-based practice essentials from the enlisted articles in bibliography.

Uterus is a muscular organ and inspects the uterine cavity having walls apposed to each other. There is a need of distension medium to widen the uterine chamber and improve visibility. This is accomplished using a variety of distension media. This preliminary study suggests that a liquid with the same viscosity as normal saline distends the uterine cavity at a pressure of approximately 40 mm Hg.

Commonly used distension media include the following ***(Fig. 1)****:*

1. *Normal saline (NS):* It is a sterile solution of sodium chloride in water. It is commonly employed as a distension medium in hysteroscopy due to its compatibility with human tissues.

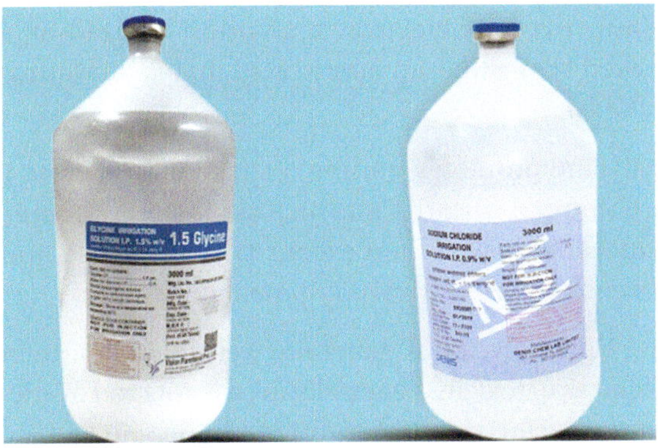

Fig. 1: Distension media.

2. *Lactated Ringer's solution:* Lactated Ringer's solution, like normal saline, is an isotonic fluid that can be utilized for distension.
3. *Dextrose solution:* A solution of dextrose (sugar) in water can be employed as a distension agent.
4. *Carbon dioxide (CO_2):* During hysteroscopy, CO_2 gas can be utilized to expand the uterus. It is absorbed by the body following the treatment reducing postoperative discomfort caused by remaining fluid when fluids are used as distension media.

CHOICE OF DISTENSION MEDIUM

It is determined by a variety of criteria, including the patient's condition, the healthcare provider's preferences, and the procedure's specific requirements. Each form of media has advantages and disadvantages in terms of safety, efficacy, and patient tolerance.

NS and glycine are routinely employed as distension medium in hysteroscopy, while they differ in important ways:

Normal Saline

Normal saline is a sterile solution of sodium chloride (salt) in water at a concentration comparable to bodily fluids.

Advantages: Isotonic means it has the same osmotic pressure as body fluids, potentially reducing the danger of excess fluid and electrolyte imbalances. NS is generally tolerated by tissues.

Disadvantages: Large amounts of NS might lead to hyponatremia (low sodium levels), especially in patients with specific medical conditions or extended treatments. The blood being miscible visibility is hampered during procedures if there is bleeding.

Glycine

It is a nonconductive, nonelectrolyte solution utilized as a distension medium in hysteroscopy. It is an amino acid that is not found naturally in physiological fluids.

Advantages: Glycine promotes uterine distension and clear visualization during hysteroscopy. It absorbs into the bloodstream more slowly than NS, which reduces the risk of fluid excess. Glycine is also nonconductive, lowering the likelihood of electrical equipment difficulties.

Disadvantages: While glycine is generally well-tolerated, there have been occasional instances of toxicity, especially in cases of fluid overload or greater absorption rates. Glycine should be avoided in people with compromised renal function because it is eliminated through the kidneys.

FLUID DELIVERY SYSTEM

In hysteroscopy, fluid under pressure is delivered to distend the uterus cavity, allowing for optimal visualization of the uterine cavity while minimizing patient pain and the risk of consequences **(Figs. 2 and 3)**. Several types of distribution methods can be used, each with its own benefits and considerations.

1. *Gravity-based systems:* The distension medium is elevated in a fluid bag or container and flows into the uterine cavity via gravity. The flow rate can be controlled by adjusting the height of the fluid bag relative to the patient. Gravity-based devices are simple and inexpensive; however, they may not provide precise control of fluid pressure or flow rate.
2. *Pressure-controlled systems:* These systems use a pump or regulator to provide distension medium to the uterine cavity at controlled pressure. This allows for more precise control over fluid pressure and flow rate, reducing the risk of overdistension and its consequences.

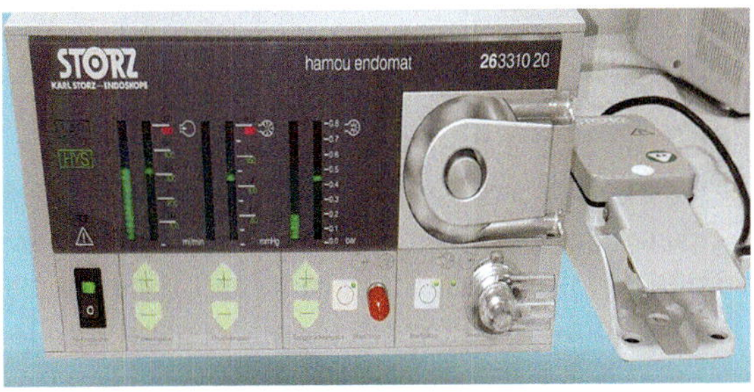

Fig. 2: Endomat.

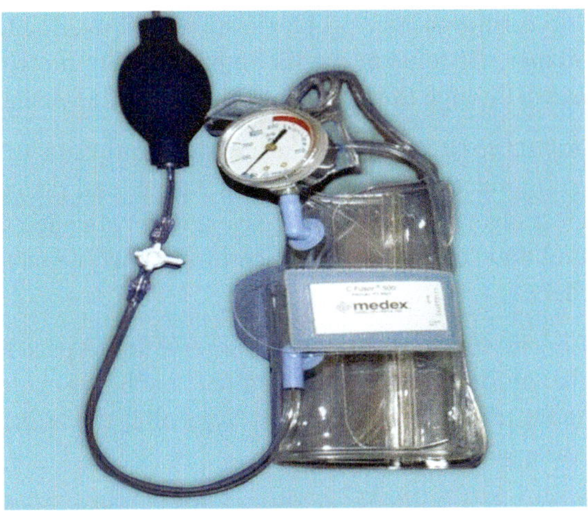

Fig. 3: Pressure bag.

Pressure-controlled systems are extensively used in modern hysteroscopy settings and can be tailored to the specific requirements of the procedure and the patient's tolerance.

3. *Integrated systems:* These systems incorporate fluid management and visualization capabilities, allowing for simultaneous irrigation and suction during hysteroscopy. These systems usually include specialized instruments with built-in irrigation and suction channels, as well as controls to regulate fluid flow and pressure. Integrated systems are convenient and efficient, allowing the surgeon to conduct a number of tasks without the need for additional or manual changes.
4. *Manual injection:* Distension medium can be injected into the uterus using a syringe or similar device. Manual injections allow the surgeon complete control over fluid distribution, but it may be less precise and take longer than automated systems.
5. *CO_2 insufflation:* During hysteroscopy, CO_2 gas, and liquid distension medium can be used to widen the uterine cavity. CO_2 insufflation systems typically employ a specialist device to inject controlled amounts of CO_2 gas into the uterine cavity, resulting in improved vision while limiting fluid absorption and associated issues.

COMPLICATIONS

Fluid overload: Excessive absorption of distension medium, especially with high volumes or lengthy procedures, can cause fluid overload. This can lead to electrolyte abnormalities, like hyponatremia (low sodium levels) or fluid overload issues.

Fluid intravasation: When distension media enters the bloodstream by uterine rupture or excessive absorption, it can cause fluid intravasation. This can lead to cardiovascular problems such fluid overload, pulmonary edema, or collapse. Distension media enter the systemic circulation by retrograde passage through the fallopian tubes and endometrium.

Electrolyte imbalances: Absorbing excessive amounts of distension media containing electrolytes, like normal saline, can cause electrolyte imbalances. Electrolyte imbalances can have a variety of effects on physical functioning, and they are especially concerning in people with underlying medical disorders.

Symptoms of persistent fluid: After the surgery, some patients may feel abdominal discomfort, bloating, or vaginal discharge from persistent distension media in the uterine cavity. Typically, these symptoms are transient and disappear on their own.

Adverse reactions: Some patients may have adverse reactions to distension media components such preservatives or additives. Allergic reactions can range from modest skin reactions to severe systemic reactions, such as anaphylaxis.

Open blood vessels and sinuses during uterine tissue resection if intrauterine pressure exceeds venous sinus or blood vessel pressure.

Factors that influence the absorption of distension fluid include:

- High intrauterine pressure leads to increased fluid absorption in the body, especially when it surpasses the mean arterial pressure. Furthermore, intrauterine pressures above 75 mm Hg increase the volume of media going back through the fallopian tubes and into the peritoneal cavity. Reduced mean artery pressure leads to reduced intrauterine pressure and fluid flow into the systemic circulation. Patients with cardiovascular co-morbidities and the elderly should exercise caution.
- Larger uterine cavities allow for better fluid absorption and require lengthier operations. However, while requiring more implanted fluid, high intrauterine pressures that allow optimal visualization are more difficult to attain.
- *Depth of myometrial penetration:* If tissue injury spreads into the deeper myometrium, fluid can be quickly absorbed by venous sinuses.
- Long duration surgery might lead to fluid accumulation within the body.

Thus, rapid systemic fluid absorption is greatest with prolonged hysteroscopic procedures using large diameter endoscopes with high rates of media inflow creating significantly elevated intrauterine pressure and where uterine trauma and vessel transection occur such as with hysteroscopic myomectomy especially FIGO type I/II fibroids, metroplasty and endometrial resection. To lessen the risk of these complications healthcare providers closely monitor patients during hysteroscopy, alter the volume and composition of the distension media as needed, and respond timely to any issues that emerge during or after the surgery. Additionally, following sterile methods and correct instrument sterilization protocols can help reduce the risk of infection.

ENERGY SOURCES USED IN OPERATIVE HYSTEROSCOPY

Electrosurgery uses high-frequency current to cut, coagulate, or vaporize tissue. It is one of the most often utilized energy sources in hysteroscopy and can be supplied in a variety of ways, including bipolar and monopolar.

Bipolar Electrosurgery

- Bipolar electrosurgery uses two closely spaced electrodes on the same instrument. The electrical current solely flows through the tissue between the two electrodes, reducing the possibility of unintentional harm to neighboring tissues.

  Since it uses two electrodes close together, the chance of tissue damage compared to monopolar electrosurgery is low. The electrical current only flows through the tissue between the two electrodes, producing more specific tissue effects.

- *PROS of bipolar electrosurgery:* Reduced chance of unintentional tissue damage and the ability to use without a grounding pad, which reduces the danger of skin burns and electrical injuries.
- Reduced chance of electrical interference with surrounding electronic equipment.

Monopolar Electrosurgery

Monopolar electrosurgery utilizes an active electrode to provide high-frequency electrical current to target organ. The electrical current flows through the tissue to a grounding pad on the patient's body, completing the circuit.

Advantages:

- Effective for cutting and coagulating tissues.
- Provides deeper tissue penetration and a larger thermal effect than bipolar electrosurgery.
- Supports various electrode shapes and sizes for surgical applications.

Considerations:

- Danger of accidental tissue injury, including heat damage to neighboring structures.
- Requires a grounding pad, which can raise the danger of skin burns and electrical injuries if not correctly put or monitored.
- Risk of electrical interference with surrounding electronic equipment.

Bipolar Resectoscope

A bipolar resectoscope is comparable to a monopolar resectoscope, however it has a different energy delivery method. A bipolar resectoscope typically contains the following components **(Fig. 4)**:

- *Scope:* Similar to a monopolar resectoscope, the scope is a slender, elongated tube with an optical system (camera) at one end for visualization of the uterus.
- The working element of a bipolar resectoscope refers to the electrode or wire loop utilized for cutting or coagulation. It is inserted through a passage in the scope and can be controlled by the surgeon to execute a variety of surgical procedures.
- The sheath protects the functional element and guides it into the uterine cavity.
- *Bipolar electrodes:* Unlike monopolar resectoscopes, which need a separate grounding pad, bipolar resectoscopes have two closely spaced electrodes in the same instrument. These electrodes provide electrical

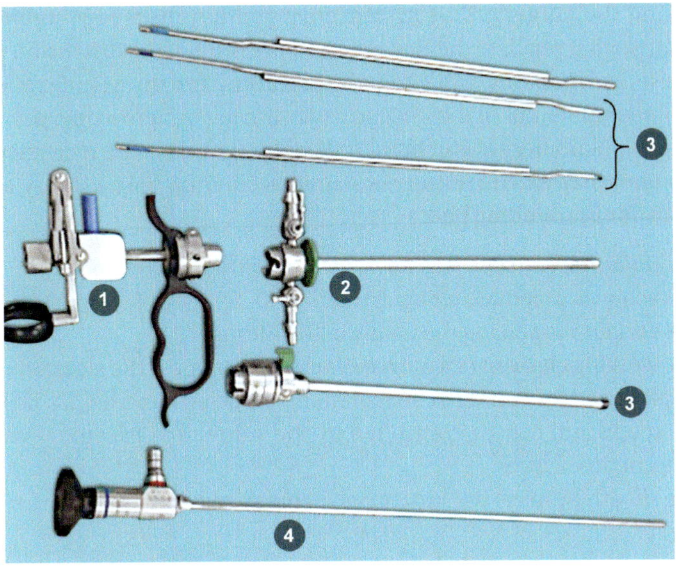

Fig. 4: Parts of resectoscope. (1) Working element; (2) Outer sheath; (3) Inner sheath; (4) Telescope.

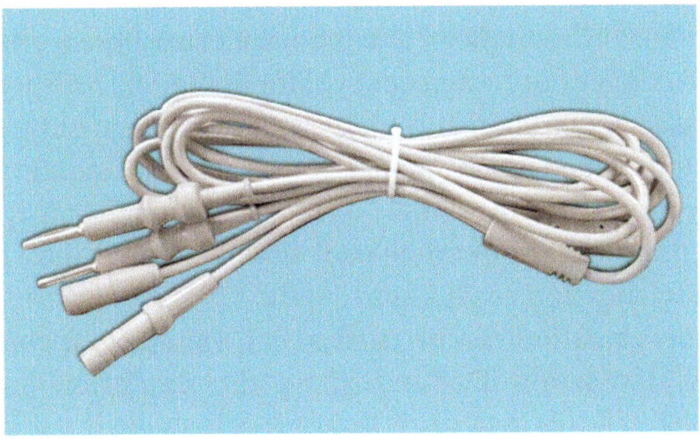

Fig. 5: Bipolar electrode cable.

current directly to the target tissue, lowering the chance of unintentional tissue damage when compared to monopolar resectoscopes.

- *Connect to the bipolar electrosurgical unit (ESU):* A bipolar resectoscope is attached to a specialized bipolar ESU, which supplies the electrical current required for cutting or coagulation. The bipolar ESU generates an electrical current between the resectoscope's two electrodes, resulting in a regulated energy field that solely affects the tissue between the electrodes **(Fig. 5)**.
- *Fluid management system:* Both monopolar and bipolar resectoscopes use a fluid management system to irrigate and dilate the uterine cavity

during the surgery. This system may contain fluid bags, tubing, and controls that regulate the flow rate and pressure of the distension media.

These components work together to allow for the visualization and surgical manipulation of the uterine cavity during hysteroscopic procedures that use bipolar energy. The bipolar design minimizes the risks associated with monopolar electrosurgery, such as accidental tissue injury and the necessity for a grounding pad.

A monopolar resectoscope is often made up of multiple components:

- The scope is a slender, elongated tube with an optical system (camera) at one end for visualizing the inside of the uterus.
- The working element of a monopolar resectoscope is the electrode or wire loop utilized for cutting or coagulation. It is inserted through a passage in the scope and can be controlled by the surgeon to execute a variety of surgical procedures.
- The sheath protects the functional element and guides it into the uterine cavity.
- *Connecting to an ESU:* A monopolar resectoscope requires an ESU to supply electrical current for cutting or coagulation procedures **(Fig. 6)**. ESU usually has controls for altering the power settings and modes of operation.

  In conclusion, monopolar and bipolar electrosurgery offer advantages and disadvantages in hysteroscopy. Monopolar electrosurgery provides deeper tissue penetration and a larger thermal effect, but it is more likely to cause unintended tissue damage and requires a grounding pad. Bipolar electrosurgery lowers the danger of accidental tissue damage and can be performed without a grounding pad, although it may have limitations in cutting efficiency and coagulation depth.
- *Laser:* Laser radiation can be used to cut, vaporize, or coagulate tissue during hysteroscopy. Depending on the operation and surgeon's

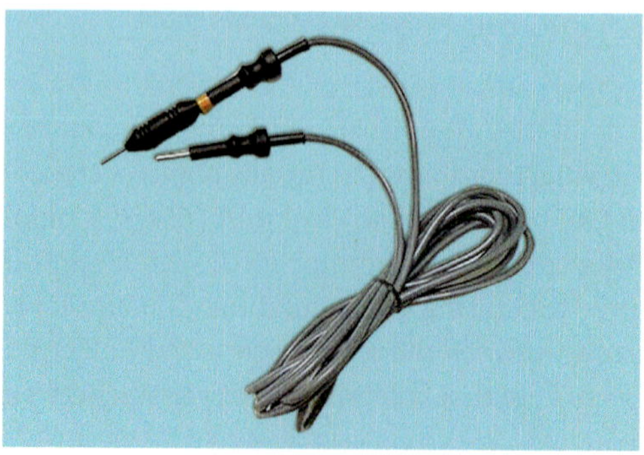

Fig. 6: Monopolar electrode cable.

preferences, many lasers, including Nd:YAG (Neodymium-doped yttrium aluminum garnet) and CO_2, can be employed. Laser energy provides precise tissue engagement, which is especially valuable for operations that need precision control and little thermal spread.

- *Mechanical energy sources*, such as tissue-cutting devices or morcellators, can be employed to remove tissue during hysteroscopy. These devices are especially beneficial for removing bigger tissue masses or polyps from the uterine cavity while causing minimal harm to adjacent tissues. Intrauterine Bigatti shaver was used. This device used a mechanical rotational cutting power with no electrical current.
- *Ultrasonic energy:* Ultrasonic shears or harmonic scalpels can be used to cut and coagulate tissue during hysteroscopy. Ultrasound energy causes mechanical vibrations that breakdown tissue while also coagulating blood vessels, resulting in accurate tissue dissection with little heat injury.
- *Radiofrequency energy* can be utilized for tissue ablation, coagulation, or vaporization during hysteroscopy. Radiofrequency energy devices create heat within the tissue, causing coagulation and vaporization of the target tissue while minimizing injury to other tissues.

The choice of energy source is determined by a number of criteria, including the procedure's precise aims, the kind of tissue being treated, and the surgeon's experience and preferences. Each energy source has distinct advantages and disadvantages in terms of tissue contact, precision, safety, and cost.

In hysteroscopy, both monopolar and bipolar electrosurgery are commonly used energy sources for cutting, coagulation, and vaporization of tissue. Here is a comparison between the two:

The surgeon's experience and preference, as well as the exact goals of the treatment and the type of tissue being treated, all influence the decision between the two.

SUGGESTED READING

1. Ansari SH, Bigatti G, Aghssa MM. Operative hysteroscopy with the Bigatti shaver (IBS®) for the removal of placental remnants. Facts Views Vis Obgyn. 2018;10(3):153-9.
2. Baker VL, Adamson GD. Intrauterine pressure and uterine distention. J Am Assoc Gynecol Laparosc. 1996;3(Suppl 4):S3.
3. Baker VL, Adamson GD. Minimum intrauterine pressure required for uterine distention. J Am Assoc Gynecol Laparosc. 1998;5(1):51-3.
4. Colacurci N, De Franciscis P, Mollo A, Litta P, Perino A, Cobellis L, et al. Small-diameter hysteroscopy with Versapoint versus resectoscopy with a unipolar knife for the treatment of septate uterus: a prospective randomized study. J Minim Invasive Gynecol. 2007;14(5):622–7.

5. Corson SL. Hysteroscopic fluid management. J Am Assoc Gynecol Laparosc. 1997;4(3):375-9.
6. Garuti G, Luerti M. Hysteroscopic bipolar surgery: a valuable progress or a technique under investigation? Curr Opin Obstet Gynecol. 2009;21(4):329-34.
7. Huser M, Papíková Z, Dziakova M, Hudeček R, Ventruba P. Radiofrequency endometrial ablation: new possibility of heavy menstrual bleeding conservative treatment. Ceska Gynekol. 2018;83(6):418-23.
8. Kulkarni AV, Kulkarni VM, Alahabade R, Ruikar PD, Mahajan R, Kulkarni T, et al. Hysteroscopic Metroplasty using Holmium: YAG Laser for Treatment of Septate Uterus. J Minim Invasive Gynecol. 2024;31(4):271-2.
9. Liu W, Yue Y, Hou X, Han H, Wang W, Lin X. Combined hysteroscopic Bigatti shaver (IBS) and resectoscope removal of a heterotopic cesarean scar pregnancy in the first trimester. Fertil Steril. 2024;122(3):546-8.
10. Vulgaropulos SP, Haley LC, Hulka JF. Intrauterine pressure and fluid absorption during continuous flow hysteroscopy. Am J Obstet Gynecol. 1992;167(2):386-90; discussion 390-91.

3

CHAPTER

Vaginoscopy: Method of Hysteroscopy

Manoj Chellani

INTRODUCTION

Hysteroscopy word is originated from Latin word "haustera," i.e., womb. In the current scenario, hysteroscopy has become the gold standard while assessing the vagina, cervix, cervical canal, and uterine cavity. It is the method of observing and operating in the endometrial cavity from a transcervical approach, offering the benefit of direct visualization of the uterine cavity while giving the option of collecting histological biopsy samples under visual control. Ambulatory hysteroscopy is a safe, feasible, and accurate method for diagnosing intrauterine pathology and treating numerous intrauterine, endocervical complications.[1,2] It can be used for the evaluation of the uterine cavity in cases of abnormal uterine bleeding (AUB), infertility, and recurrent pregnancy loss. The technique of the vaginal hysteroscopy (VH) or office diagnostic hysteroscopy is different from the standard technique. Vaginal hysteroscopy now widely used globally due to its convenience as it does not require anesthesia use, and success in evaluating the uterine cavity.[3] However, still this technique not used by many clinicians due to having lesser experience in performing the procedure. But clinician doctors should be familiar with both standard hysteroscopy and vaginoscopy in the office setting.[4] Diagnostic hysteroscopy is performed using two different techniques:

Traditional Technique

A Sims speculum inserted into the vagina to visualize the cervix, and a vulsellum is applied to the anterior lip of uterine cervix to create countertraction to facilitate the insertion of the hysteroscope. For the distension of the vagina, cervical canal, and uterine cavity, 0.9% normal saline solution is used in both diagnostic and surgical hysteroscopy.

Vaginoscopy (No-touch Technique)

Vaginoscopy is known as "No-touch" technique. It is an alternative technique, where hysteroscope is first introduced into the introitus of the vagina and avoids the use of the speculum and a tenaculum to grasp or steady the cervix

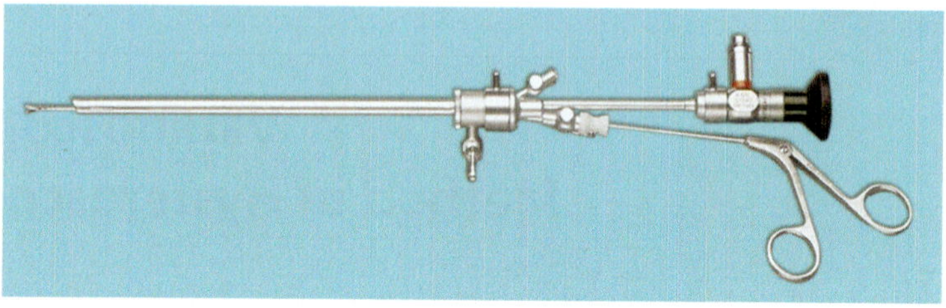

Fig. 1: Hysteroscopy.

(Fig. 1) (Busquets, CLARK). The vagina is then distended with the saline distention medium and hysteroscope directed toward the cervix, the cervical canal, and then into the uterine cavity.[5,6]

The vaginoscopy approach was first described by Bettocchi and Selvaggi in 1997.[7,8] Since then, this method has been used for a wide variety of applications. Within the pediatric and adolescent population, vaginoscopy is perform to evaluate and treat various conditions including abnormal uterine bleeding, retained products of conception, endometrial polyps, and for identification of distorted anatomy.[9,10] Its use has also been documented in the treatment of vaginal lesions and for diagnosis of cervical dysplasia.[11,12] In the field of urogynecology, vaginoscopy has also been used to identify mesh erosion more successfully[7,13] and has also been used for the evaluation of fistula formation.[14]

METHODS OF VAGINOSCOPY

Informed Consent

The hospital staff first ask some questions (name, age, allergies any other complications) to patients. After that, staff/doctor should inform to the patients through each step of procedure. After that a consent form should be sign with patients and her guardian before the procedure. After signing the consent form, patients should be shift to operation theater.

Insertion of Vaginoscope and Examination

The vaginoscope is gently insert through the vulva, vagina, and then the cervical canal, using normal saline to dilate the front of the scope without prior dilation. During the insertion of the vaginoscope, patients may expect to experience little to no discomfort. After insertion of the vaginoscope the cervical canal can be examine for polypi, Nabothian cysts or micropolypi that indicate chronic cervicitis. The best view of the entire uterine cavity is obtained when the hysteroscope is place at the junction of the lower uterine segment and the upper cervical canal. The uterine cavity can be systematically starting from its anterior and posterior walls, fundus, and borders, and the examination is considered complete if both tubal ostia are reached, describing any gross pathology, such as septum, adhesions, polyp, myoma, growths, etc.[3,15]

In addition to procedure, to decrease pain and improve comfort for patients, patients can be administered lorazepam prior to the procedure to decrease anxiety and nervousness.

The addition of music therapy has been shown to calm patients and promote comfort during the procedure.

Pain can be reduced by performing a paracervical block prior to the procedure, administering lidocaine in the hysteroscopy fluid, and prescribing nonsteroidal anti-inflammatory drugs (NSAIDs) for postoperative cramps and pain.

Additionally, this procedure can be conduct in an outpatient setting which can ultimately be more convenient and cost effective for patients.

The five steps for vaginoscopy:

1. Introducing the scope into the vagina
2. Guiding the scope into the posterior vaginal fornix
3. Identifying the external cervical os and introducing the scope to the canal
4. Following the cervical canal to enter the uterine cavity
5. Evaluation of the uterine cavity

TECHNICAL SPECIFICATIONS OF LIGHT SOURCE

Hysteroscopy procedure always performed under videoendoscopic control, therefore the cold light source has a major effect on image quality. A high-quality cold light source, preferably equipped with a Xenon lamp, typically yield the best outcomes. Commonly, a 175-watt light source is appropriate for routine procedures, whereas for special applications or those performed with miniature telescopes, a 300-watt light source recommended. Operating a light source at higher power levels typically results in the generation of more thermal energy, leading to a greater increase in temperature. Light is transmitted through fiber-optic or fluid light cables measuring 3.5–5 mm in diameter and ranging from 180 to 350 cm in length, while standard hysteroscopic procedures use cold light cables that are 5 mm in diameter and 180 cm in length.[16]

BENEFITS

Vaginoscopy offers numerous advantages over traditional hysteroscopy, including reduced discomfort, shorter procedure and recovery times, fewer vasovagal events, and enhanced visualization of structures. This procedure can be performed by surgeons in an outpatient setting or in the operating room with conscious sedation or general anesthesia, potentially leading to increased patient satisfaction and serving as a substitute for standard hysteroscopy in outpatient settings.

USE OF VAGINOSCOPY IN INFERTILITY TREATMENT

The advantages of routine use of outpatient vaginoscopy over traditional hysteroscopy in a randomized control trial of over 1500 women in the United Kingdom indicated decreased patient pain, shorter procedural times, higher rates of success, and easier maneuverability for the clinicians.[17] A recent comprehensive review, which incorporated six randomized control trials of outpatient vaginoscopy, recommended that this technique becomes the standard of care for office hysteroscopy, as it is faster, less painful, and less likely to induce a vasovagal reaction.[18] The AAGL and ACOG both advocate for considering the use of vaginoscopy for outpatient hysteroscopy.[19] Additionally, the French College of Gynecologists and Obstetricians has endorsed vaginoscopy as the standard of care for diagnostic hysteroscopy since 2014.[20]

USE IN EXAMINATION OF CHILDREN

Vaginoscopy is commonly used to examine children, allowing the clinician to select an instrument that would not harm the hymen or lower genital tract of the nonestrogenized child. This method emphasizes the significance of maintaining anatomical integrity of the child's hymenal tissue for cultural and forensic purposes, as families often seek assurance that vaginoscopy preserves the child's sexual abstinence while anatomic disruptions of the hymenal tissues might serve as forensic evidence of childhood sexual abuse.[21]

COMPARISON OF VAGINOSCOPE VERSUS STANDARD HYSTEROSCOPE

Most of the previous studies reported less pain in vaginoscopy than in standard hysteroscopy **(Table 1)**.[4,17,22-24] However, Sharma et al.[25] observed no differences in pain scores between vaginoscopy and standard hysteroscopy. In retrospective study, there are no significant differences in the success rates between the vaginoscopy and standard hysteroscopy groups. However, vaginoscopy had shorter procedural time and caused lesser pain than the standard hysteroscopy. Moreover, the postoperative complication and infection rates were not increase in vaginoscopy.[4]

TABLE 1: Pain score (VAS) in vaginoscope and standard hysteroscope.

S. no	*Studied by*	*Vaginoscopy*	*Standard hysteroscopy*	*p value*
1.	Tien et al., 2021	3 (maximum of 10)	5 (maximum of 10)	$p = 0.01$
2.	Smith et al., 2019	42.7 (maximum of 100)	42.7 (maximum of 100)	$p = 0.02$
3.	Almeida et al., 2008	1.60 (maximum of 10)	3.39 (maximum of 10)	$p = 0.01$
4.	Garbin et al., 2006	0.5 (maximum of 10)	2 (maximum of 10)	$p < 0.001$
5.	Sagiv et al., 2006	3.8 (maximum of 10)	5.3 (maximum of 10)	$p = 0.008$

A randomized case control study reported the significantly lower mean-time is required for the procedures of vaginoscopy (4.44 ± 1.050 minutes) as compared to the traditional hysteroscopy (5.71 ± 1.209 minutes). The time taken to perform complete hysteroscopy was significantly shorter with vaginoscopy hysteroscopy.[3] In another study also reported that the lesser procedural time required in vaginoscopy group as compared to the standard hysteroscopy group (median time, 135 vs. 190 seconds). The time taken for the examination varied between the different hysteroscopy methods, with the hysteroscopy group taking the longest time compared to the vaginoscopy group ($p < 0.01$). The VAS scores immediately after the examination and 30 minutes after the examination were both significantly higher in the hysteroscopy group than in the vaginoscopy group ($p < 0.01$).[26]

A retrospective cohort study reported that the difference in pain stress response indices [levels of neuropeptide (NPY), prostaglandin E2 (PGE2) and 5-hydroxytryptamine (5-HT)] after the pain-causing mediator intervention was significantly better in the vaginoscopy group as compared to hysteroscopy group. The difference in the incidence of complications such as abortion syndrome, cervical laceration, uterine perforation, and hemorrhage after treatment was significantly lesser in the vaginoscopy group as compared to hysteroscopy group. In the vaginoscopy group, the satisfaction rate was 91% significantly higher as compared to the hysteroscopy group ($p < 0.05$).[26]

CONCLUSION

Vaginoscopy procedure requires less examination time and less recovery time, and involved lower pain as compared to the standard hysteroscopy. However, both techniques have similar success rates. The vaginoscopy procedure has been shown to better visualization of the vaginal canal, cervix, and uterine cavity therefore, it is a good option for office hysteroscopic examinations. Moreover, this technique provides an alternative method for patients, particularly in sexual abstinence women or girls.

REFERENCES

1. Clark TJ, Voit D, Gupta JK, et al. Accuracy of hysteroscopy in the diagnosis of endometrial cancer and hyperplasia: a systematic quantitative review. JAMA. 2002;288(13):1610-21. DOI: 10.1001/jama.288.13.1610.
2. Jacobs I, Tibosch R, Geomini P, Coppus S, Bongers MY, van Hanegem N. Atypical endometrial polyps and the incidence of endometrial cancer: a retrospective cohort study. BJOG. 2020;127(8):994-9. doi: 10.1111/1471-0528.16194.
3. Gupta N, Jahan U, Yadav A, et al. Comparative evaluation of vaginoscopic vs. traditional hysteroscopy. World J Lap Surg. 2021;14(2):98-102.
4. Tien CT, Li PC, Ding DC. Outcome comparison between vaginoscopy and standard hysteroscopy: a retrospective cohort study. J Chin Med Assoc. 2021;84(5):536-9.

5. Busquets M, Lemus M. Practicability of panoramic hysteroscopy with CO_2, Clinical experience: 923 cases. Rev Chil Obstet Ginecol. 1993;58(2): 113-8. Spanish. PMID: 8209037.3.
6. Clark TJ, Gupta JK. Handbook of outpatient hysteroscope: a complete guide to diagnosis and therapy, 1st edition. London: Hodder Education; 2005.
7. Bettocchi S, Nappi L, Ceci O, Selvaggi L. Office hysteroscopy. Obstet Gynecol Clin North Am. 2004;31(3):641-54.
8. Darwish AM, Youssef AA. Screening sonohysterography in infertility. Gynecol Obstet Invest. 1999;48(1):43-7.
9. Darwish AM, Sayed EH, Mohammad SA, Mohammad II, Hassan HI. Reliability of out-patient hysteroscopy in one-stop clinic for abnormal uterine bleeding. Gynecologic Surgery. 2012;9(3):289-95.
10. Emanuel MH. New developments in hysteroscopy. Best Pract Res Clin Obstet Gynaecol. 2013;pii:S1521-6934(13)00005-9.
11. Eimers JM, te Velde ER, Gerritse R, van Kooy RJ, Kremer J, Habbema JD. The validity of the postcoital test for estimating the probability of conceiving. Am J Obstet Gynecol. 1994;171(1):65-70.
12. Dechaud H, Daures JP, Hedon B. Prospective evaluation of falloposcopy. Hum Reprod. 1998;13:1815-8.
13. Glatstein IZ, Sleeper LA, Lavy Y, Simon A, Adoni A, Palti Z, Hurwitz A, Laufer N. Observer variability in the diagnosis and management of hysterosalpingogram. Fertil Steril. 1997;67:223-37.
14. Kessler I, Lancet M. Hysterography and hysteroscopy: a comparison. Fertil Steril. 1986;46:709-10.
15. Darwish AM, Hassanin AI, Aleem MAA, et al. Routine vaginoscopic office hysteroscopy in modern infertility work-up: a randomized controlled trial. Gynecol Surg. 2014;11:185-9. https://doi.org/10.1007/s10397-014-0840-x.
16. Luca Mencaglia, Luiz Cavalcanti De Albuquerque Neto, R. Alfonso Arias Alvarez. Manual of hysteroscopy: diagnostic, operative and office hysteroscopy. Hysteroscopy. 2013; Endo Press, p. 11.
17. Smith PP, Kolhe S, O'Connor S, Clark TJ. Vaginoscopy against standard treatment: a randomised controlled trial. BJOG. 2019;126:891-9.
18. de Silva PM, Carnegy A, Smith PP, et al. Vaginoscopy for office hysteroscopy: a systematic review and meta-analysis. Eur J Obstet Gynecol Reprod Biol. 2020;252:278-85.
19. The use of hysteroscopy for the diagnosis and treatment of intrauterine pathology. ACOG Committee opinion, number 800. Obstetrics and Gynecology. 2020;135:e138-48.
20. Deffieux X, Gauthier T, Menager N, et al. Hysteroscopy: Guidelines for clinical practice from the French College of Gynaecologists and Obstetricians. EJOG. 2014;178:114-22.
21. Desar S, Namazi G, Nahas S, Stuparich M, Behbehani S. To visualize beyond: Vaginoscopy. American Journal of Obstetrics and Gynecology. 2024;230(4):S1287.
22. Almeida ZMMC, Pontes R, Costa HLFF. Evaluation of pain in diagnostic hysteroscopy by vaginoscopy using normal saline at body temperature as distension medium: a randomized controlled trial. Rev Bras Ginecol Obstet. 2008;30:25-30.

23. Garbin O, Kutnahorsky R, Göllner JL, Vayssiere C. Vaginoscopic versus conventional approaches to outpatient diagnostic hysteroscopy: a two-centre randomized prospective study. Hum Reprod. 2006;21:2996-3000.
24. Sagiv R, Sadan O, Boaz M, Dishi M, Schechter E, Golan A. A new approach to office hysteroscopy compared with traditional hysteroscopy: a randomized controlled trial. Obstet Gynecol. 2006;108:387-92.
25. Sharma M, Taylor A, di Spiezio Sardo A, Buck L, Mastrogamvrakis G, Kosmas I, et al. Outpatient hysteroscopy: traditional versus the 'no-touch' technique. BJOG. 2005;112:963-7.
26. Liao L, Peng Y, Lu J, Wang Z, Xu J, Chen X, Chen H, Zhang X. Effect of vaginoscopy versus conventional hysteroscopy on pain, complications, and patient satisfaction in patients with endometrial polyps. Comput Math Methods Med. 2022:3835941. doi: 10.1155/2022/3835941.

4

CHAPTER

Office Hysteroscopy: Principles

Deepti Gupta

BACKGROUND

One of the safe, effective, well-tolerated outpatient procedures for diagnosing and managing many intrauterine pathologies is "Office Hysteroscopy." This procedure is largely independent of hospital circuits and can help minimize complications associated with general anesthesia/locoregional anesthesia.[1]

HISTORY AND EVOLUTION

The first diagnostic and operative hysteroscopic procedure is said to have been performed by Pantaleoni in 1869.[2] Adjacent functional channel was introduced by Mikulicz-Radecki and Freund in 1927 followed by use of hysteroscope with two channels by Silander in 1962. Mohri is said to have made first flexible hysteroscope in 1971, however first "operative" office hysteroscope was introduced by Bettocchi in 1996.[2]

INDICATIONS AND CONTRAINDICATIONS

- Diagnosis and management of abnormal uterine bleeding and postmenopausal bleeding
- Diagnosis and management of endometrial polyps, submucosal fibroids, and thickened endometrium
- Diagnose and remove intrauterine lesions or foreign bodies like intrauterine devices (IUDs), adhesions, retained products of conception (POCs), or uterine septum

EQUIPMENT AND INSTRUMENTATION

For diagnostic hysteroscopy, the Bettocchi office hysteroscope with a 2-mm diameter endoscope, single flow and 3.6 mm outer sheath is used whereas for both diagnostic and operative purposes, the Bettocchi Integrated Office Hysteroscope (BIOH) with a diameter of 4 mm is used.[3] With advent of smaller 5-Fr operative instruments, many procedures can be completed in office setting. Another key development was the introduction of a versatile bipolar

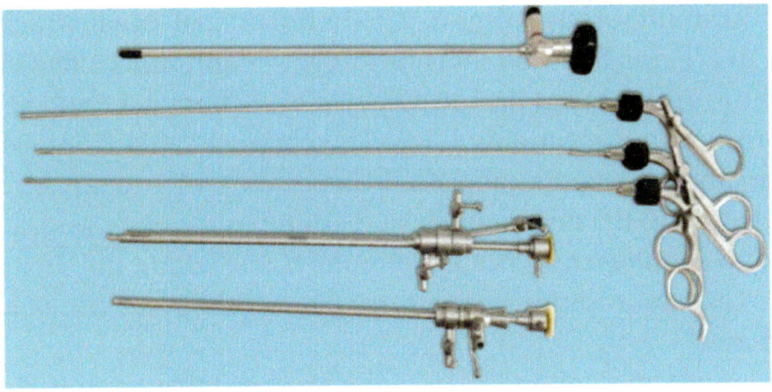

Fig. 1: Rigid office hysteroscope.

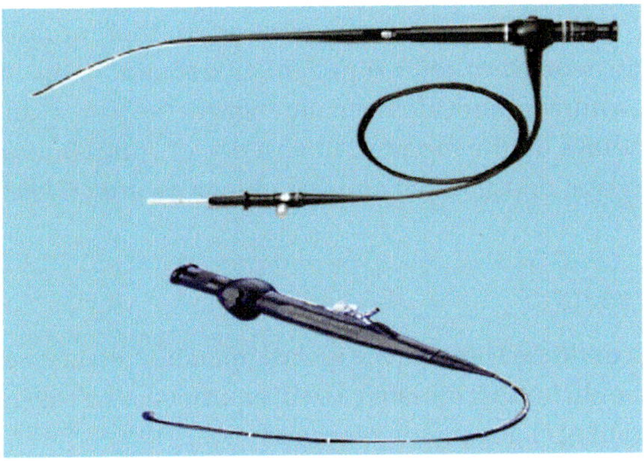

Fig. 2: A flexible office hysteroscope.

electrosurgery system in 1997 dedicated to hysteroscopy, the Gynecare VersaPoint. The use of 5-Fr bipolar electrodes has reduced the use of the resectoscope and the operating room to a smaller number of cases by making management of most pathologies possible using office hysteroscope.[4]

Rigid hysteroscopes allow for vaginoscopy and more durable operative procedures **(Fig. 1)**. Flexible hysteroscopes offer the ability to visually navigate sharp angles without contacting sensitive cervical Walls **(Fig. 2)**. However, they lack the advantage of vaginoscopy.

TECHNIQUE

Direct vaginoscopic approach is now recommended for use. Tips for surpassing/negotiating internal cervical os include:

Analgesia/Anesthesia

External cervical os is often circular in a nulliparous woman ranging from 4 to 6 mm in width and usually transverse ranging from 10 to 15 mm in width in multiparous woman. The endocervical canal which ranges from 2.5 to 3 cm is lined by folds forming a longitudinal ridge along the median line. This median line also known as "arbor vitae" and secondary crests form upward extending folds. The cervical canal is innervated by both sympathetic and parasympathetic fibers.[5] Sensitive innervations of the uterus originate in the myometrium and extend to the outer serosal surface, whereas the endometrium and any fibrotic tissue within the cavity are not sensitive. Thus, procedures can be carried out without the use of analgesia or anesthesia.[6]

In a retrospective cohort study, it was observed that approximately 80% of individuals undergoing the procedure reported a pain score of 0, while the remainder reported mild (VAS scores of 1–3) or moderate (VAS scores 4–7) discomfort.[7] It is, therefore, recommended that nonpharmacologic methods may be used to reduce patient anxiety and pain, such as "vocal local," where a nurse or provider verbally engages the patient and shows them operative findings on the monitor. In absence of contraindication, patients may be given oral nonsteroidal anti-inflammatory drug (NSAID) before the procedure.

ADVANTAGES[8]

- It can be conducted outside the formal operation theater setting
- Rooms should be appropriately sized, equipped, and staffed
- Only adjoining changing room needed
- Less invasive as bypass need for cervical dilatation
- Less painful
- Quick recovery time
- Increased cost effectiveness
- Better sustainability and decreased waste as less gowning draping needed[9]

DISADVANTAGES

- Higher cost for purchase and maintenance
- Cleaning, disinfection and sterilization needs more effort and care
- Reduced image size compared to that of standard hysteroscopy
- More frail and fragile
- Slightly tedious use

CONCLUSION

Introduction of "office" hysteroscopy has made the procedure more accessible and convenient for patients, as it can be performed in the clinic without the need for anesthesia or hospitalization. According to a study by Wortman and colleagues, OH was successful in about 92–95% of the cases, without resorting to the OR.[10] The procedures were generally well tolerated too. However, despite all this, office hysteroscopy comprises only about 25% of all hysteroscopies and should be performed more often.[11]

REFERENCES

1. Mairos J, Di Martino P. Office hysteroscopy: an operative gold standard technique and an important contribution to patient safety. Gynecol Surg. 2016;13:111-4. doi: 10.1007/s10397-015-0926-0. Epub 2016 Feb 4. PMID: 27226786; PMCID: PMC4854928.
2. Tsonis O, Gkrozou F, Lavasidis L, Paschopoulos M. The history of hysteroscopy as an endoscopic method. GinPolMedProject. 2023;18 (2):1-6.
3. Kerbage Y, Rubod C, Hubert T, et al. How I do: a low-cost hysteroscopy model. Gynecol Obstet Fertil Senol. 2018;46:664-6.
4. Bettocchi S, Ceci O, Di Venere R, et al. Advanced operative office hysteroscopy without anesthesia: analysis of 501 cases treated with a 5-Fr bipolar electrode. Hum Reprod. 2002;17:2435e2438.
5. Burkitt HG, Young B, Heath JW. The female genital organs in Wheather's functional histology. Edited by Longman Group UK; 1993. pp.335-65.
6. Bettocchi S, Ceci O, Nappi L, et al. Operative office hysteroscopy without anesthesia: analysis of 4863 cases performed with mechanical instruments. J Am Gynecol Laparosc. 2004;11:59e61.
7. Telang M, Shetty TS, Puntambekar SS, Telang PM, Panchal S, Alnure Y. Three thousand cases of office hysteroscopy: see and treat an Indian experience. J Obstet Gynaecol India. 2020;70(5):384-9. https://doi.org/10.1007/s13224-020-01334-4. Epub 2020 Jul 17. PMID: 33041557; PMCID: PMC7516003.
8. Sardo ADS, Calagna G, Carlo CD. Tips and tricks in office hysteroscopy. Gynecology and Minimally Invasive Therapy. 2015;4(1):3-7. ISSN 2213-3070.
9. Wright KN, Hamilton K, Kosturakis A. An Overview of Office Hysteroscopy. Curr Obstet Gynecol Rep. 2024;13:88-96. https://doi.org/10.1007/s13669-024-00377-y.
10. Wortman M, Daggett A, Ball C. Operative hysteroscopy in an office-based surgical setting: review of Patient Safety and satisfaction in 414 cases. J Minim Invasive Gynecol. 2013;20(Issue 1):56-63.
11. Shields J, Dilday E, Chang S, Kho K. Moving hysteroscopy from the office to the operating room: a comparison of clinical outcomes and resource utilization. High Value Practice Academic Alliance National Conference;2018.

5

CHAPTER

Office Hysteroscopy in Abnormal Uterine Bleeding

Megha Karnik

Abnormal uterine bleeding (AUB) is frequently encountered in peri- and postmenopausal women during routine clinical practice. Several diagnostic modalities, including transvaginal ultrasound, hysterosalpingography, dilatation and curettage, endometrial biopsy, and endometrial aspiration, are used in the evaluation and management of AUB.[1] Over recent years, office hysteroscopy, in conjunction with endometrial biopsy or aspiration, has emerged as the primary approach for diagnosing AUB. This preference has evolved as evidence demonstrates the superiority of outpatient hysteroscopy combined with endometrial biopsy over blind dilatation and curettage, which typically requires anesthesia and incurs additional costs.

SUBMUCOUS AND INTRAMURAL MYOMAS

In most cases, intrauterine myomas remain asymptomatic until women reach the age of 35. Approximately 80% of these myomas protrude into the uterine cavity to varying degrees. Pedunculated endocavitary myomas are less common, and their extension into the cervical canal is considered rare.[2] On hysteroscopic examination, these myomas may appear regular in shape with a smooth surface and an endometrium that looks similar to the surrounding endometrial cavity **(Figs. 1A and B)**. However, in cases with extensive intracavitary growth, the apex of the fibroid may exhibit ulceration or necrosis due to compression by the endometrium. The fibroid itself may have a pearly white appearance, often presenting with multiple visible blood vessels and a multilobulated structure **(Figs. 1C and D)**.[3]

ENDOMETRIAL POLYPS

Endometrial polyps are characterized by their exophytic growth patterns and vary widely in terms of shape, size, and number. These polyps have an epithelial surface that closely resembles the surrounding endometrium. On hysteroscopic manipulation with a grasper, sessile polyps exhibit a soft texture **(Figs. 2A and B)**. Pedunculated polyps consist of a vascularized connective tissue stalk with hypertrophic vessels, and the surface is lined

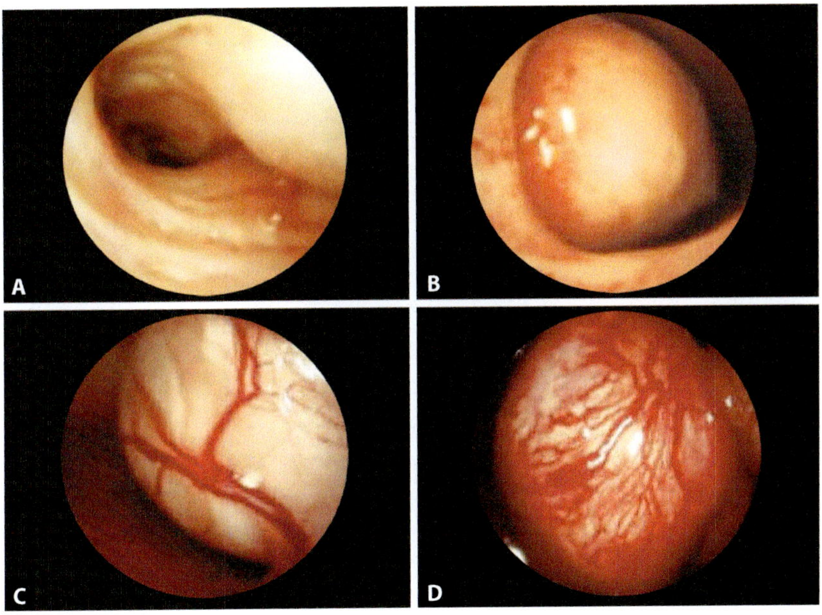

Figs. 1A to D: (A) Submucous myoma, covered by homogeneous endometrium; (B) Pedunculated myoma covered by atrophic endometrium; (C) Large blood vessel on the surface of a submucous myoma; (D) Diffuse superficial vascularization of a submucous myoma.

with cuboidal or columnar epithelium.[4] In some cases, polyps are associated with glandular hyperplasia, with long periods of latency. Since curettage has proven ineffective for the removal of polyps, they should be excised using hysteroscopic guidance to ensure complete removal and avoid recurrence. This may be possible in office hysteroscopy with analgesia depending upon patient pain tolerance **(Figs. 2C and D)**.

ENDOMETRIAL ATROPHY

Endometrial atrophy is a physiological process in postmenopausal women that can, however, cause postmenopausal bleeding. This atrophic change occurs due to hormonal fluctuations during the menopausal transition. These hormonal shifts result in the thinning of both the surface epithelium and the underlying capillaries, increasing the fragility of the stromal tissue. This condition accounts for abnormal uterine bleeding in approximately 45% of postmenopausal women who do not present with any other organic causes of bleeding.[5]

Hysteroscopically, atrophic endometrium is characterized by a thin, translucent mucosal surface through which underlying vascular patterns are often visible. Hemorrhagic suffusions and petechiae may be seen, although

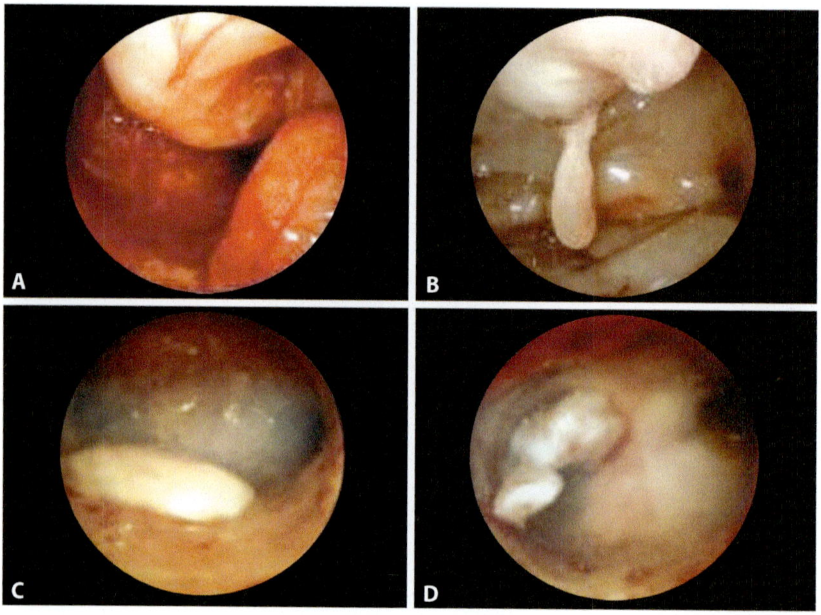

Figs. 2A to D: (A) Multiple endometrial polyps; (B) Large soft endometrial polyp; (C) Endometrial polyp located in the inferior wall of the uterus; (D) Cornual polyp cannot be removed by traditional curettage.

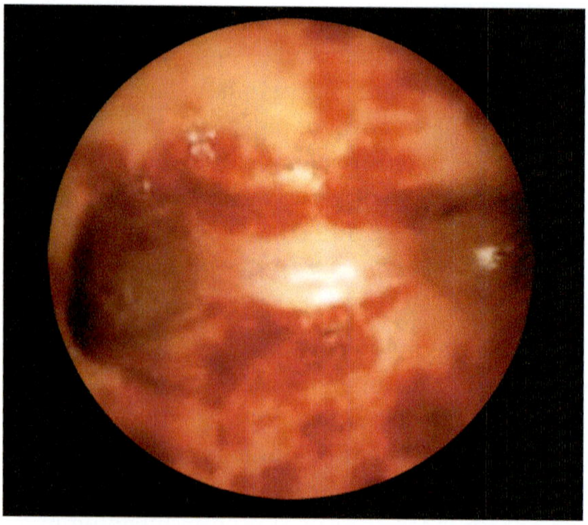

Fig. 3: Presence of diffuse hemorrhagic suffusion in menopausal patients.

these findings are typically without pathological significance **(Figs. 3 to 6)**. In cases of severe atrophy, the endometrium may take on a smooth, shiny, porcelain-like appearance.[6]

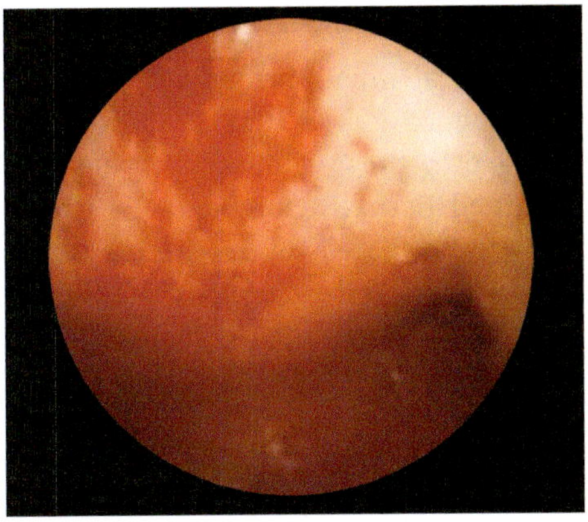

Fig. 4: Focal hemorrhagic petechiae.

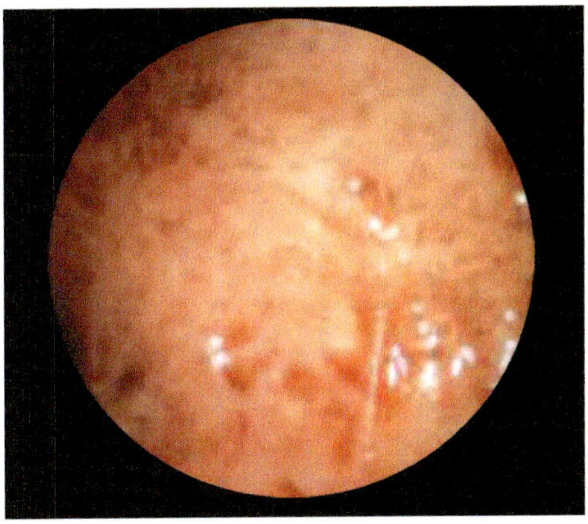

Fig. 5: Presence of endometrial varices.

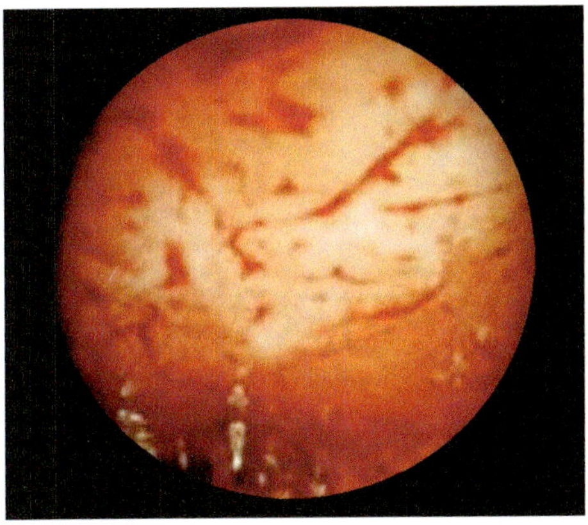

Fig. 6: Premenstrual endometrium.

POSTPARTUM METRORRHAGIA

Postpartum or postabortal bleeding can sometimes be attributed to retained products of conception (POCs) or abortive debris.[7] Diagnostic hysteroscopy is advised in these situations to ensure that the uterine cavity is free of retained tissue. Retained POCs can appear as cheesy material that adheres to focal areas of the uterine cavity **(Figs. 7 and 8)**. Removing this material under hysteroscopic guidance helps prevent complications, such as intrauterine adhesions, which are common after repeated blind curettage **(Figs. 9 and 10)**. Due to the potential for significant bleeding during the removal process, it is recommended that this procedure be performed in an operating room setting with adequate preparation for possible hemorrhage and the need for transfusion.[8]

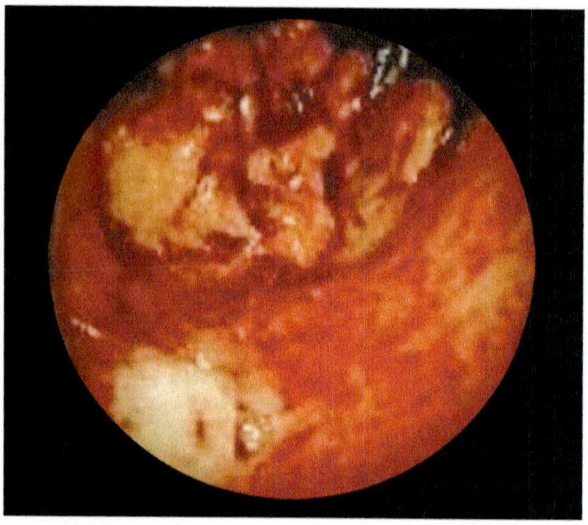

Fig. 7: Presence of abortive debris.

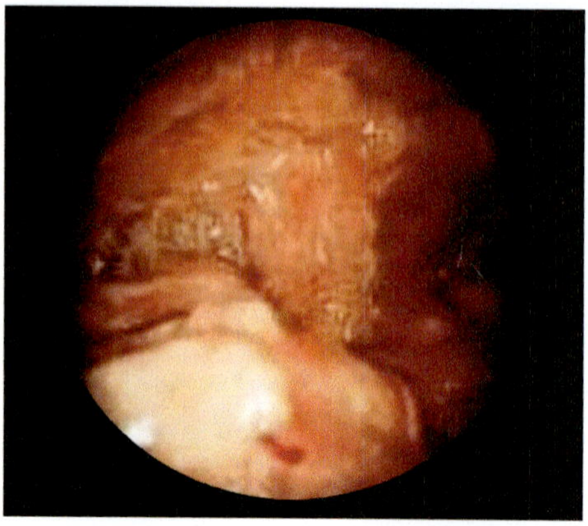

Fig. 8: Presence of abortive pregnancy.

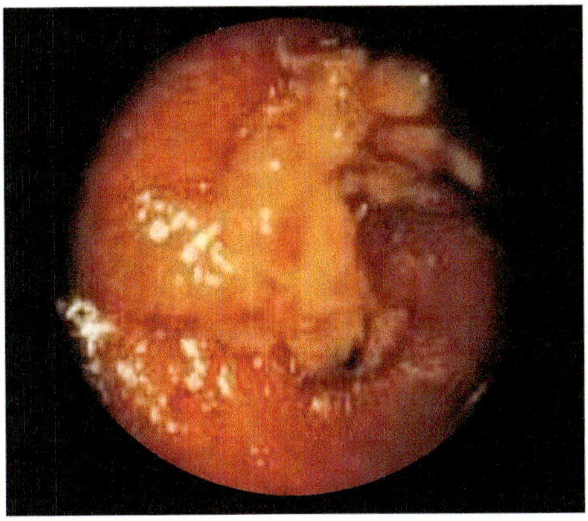

Fig. 9: Abortive debris and intrauterine synechiae.

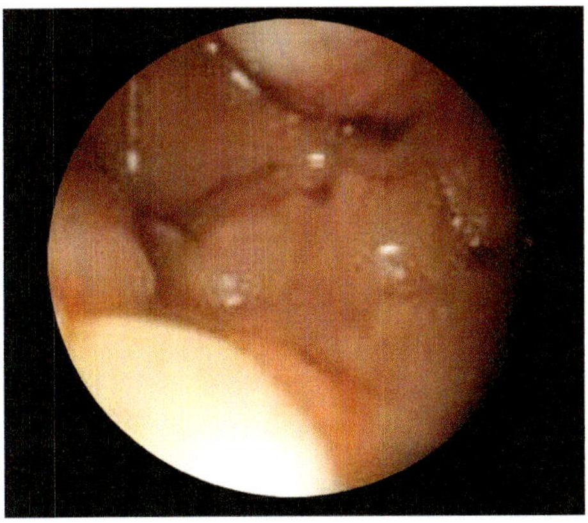

Fig. 10: After 2 weeks, incipient synechiae develops from abortion residues.

ENDOMETRIAL CARCINOMA

Endometrial hyperplasia, which is often a precursor to carcinoma, and carcinoma itself typically present with abnormal uterine bleeding. Endometrial carcinoma accounts for 8–10% of cases of postmenopausal bleeding.[9] In women presenting with AUB, the prevalence of endometrial hyperplasia is approximately 10%. Early identification and treatment of these lesions are essential to prevent the progression from hyperplasia with atypia to adenocarcinoma.

Endometrial Hyperplasia

Endometrial hyperplasia is a known precursor to endometrial carcinoma. Therefore, early detection of hyperplastic lesions in women with AUB or post-menopausal bleeding is critical.[10] Hysteroscopy allows direct visualization of the endometrial cavity and enables targeted biopsy of suspicious areas. However, not all histological aspects of endometrial hyperplasia have corresponding visual cues on hysteroscopy. Consequently, a classification system has been developed that correlates hysteroscopic findings of hyperplastic lesions with their associated risk of malignancy.

Low-risk Endometrial Hyperplasia: Hysteroscopic Aspects

Hysteroscopically, low-risk endometrial hyperplasia often resembles normal endometrium. The hysteroscope tip is used to assess the thickness of the endometrial lining, and the mucosa can display widened glandular ostia and cystic formations about 1 mm in diameter **(Figs. 11 to 13)**. In cases where similar findings are present in a thinner endometrium, this may indicate cystic atrophy. Other hysteroscopic signs

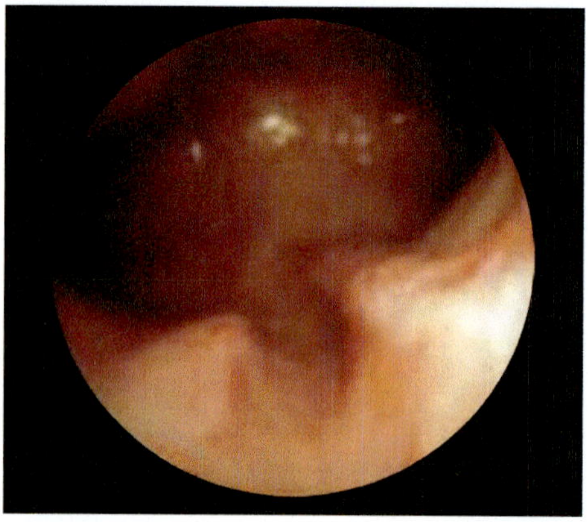

Fig. 11: Increased endometrial thickness in low-risk formations.

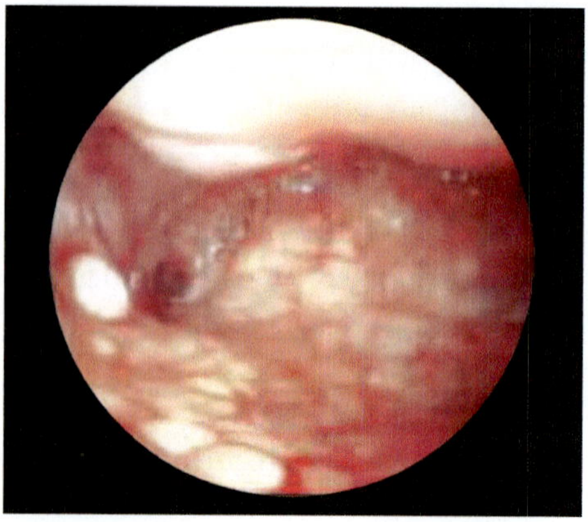

Fig. 12: Cystic glandular endometrial hyperplasia.

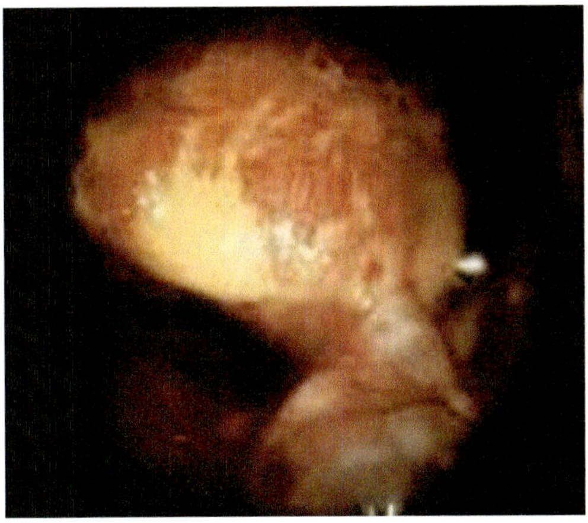

Fig. 13: Cystic atrophy.

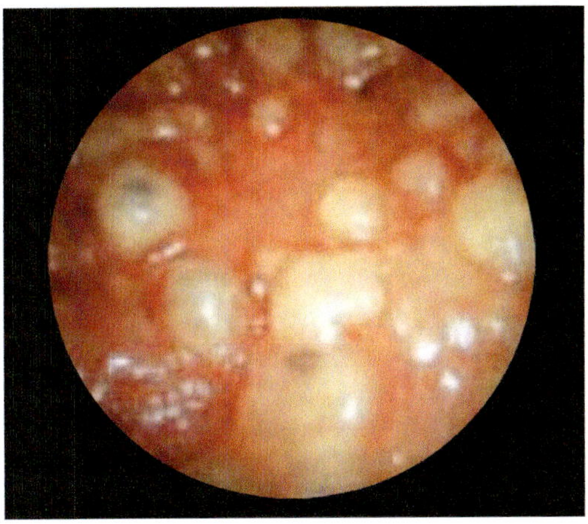

Fig. 14: Endometrial polyp with cystic formations.

that suggest low-risk hyperplasia include a thickened, nonhomogeneous endometrium, increased vascularity, polypoid appearance, and areas of cystic dilatation **(Figs. 14 to 19)**.[11]

High-risk Endometrial Hyperplasia Hysteroscopic Aspects

High-risk endometrial hyperplasia has neoplastic features, both on hysteroscopy and histopathology.[12] Hysteroscopically, the endometrium appears polypoidal, and abnormal vascularization is frequently observed, often in the form of corkscrew or tree-like patterns **(Figs. 20 to 22)**. These features should be noted, as they raise suspicion for premalignant or malignant transformation.

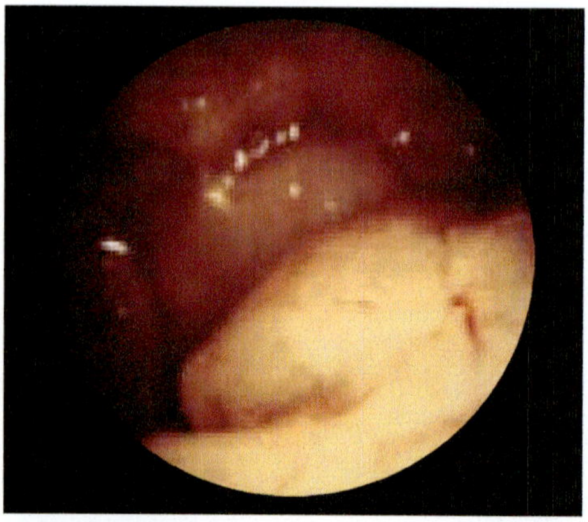

Fig. 15: Nonhomogeneous endometrial growth.

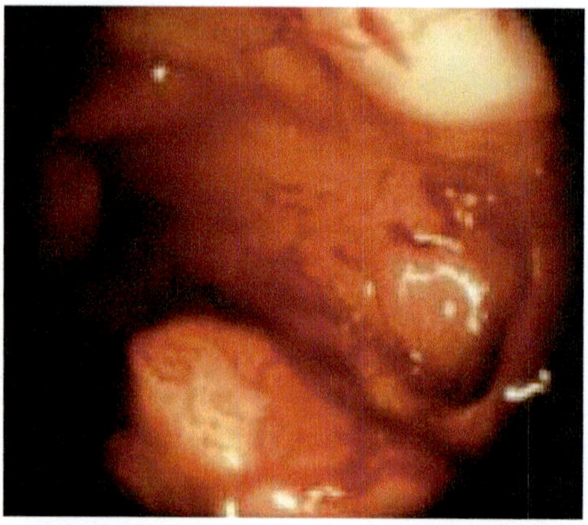

Fig. 16: Polypoid formation and increased vascularization.

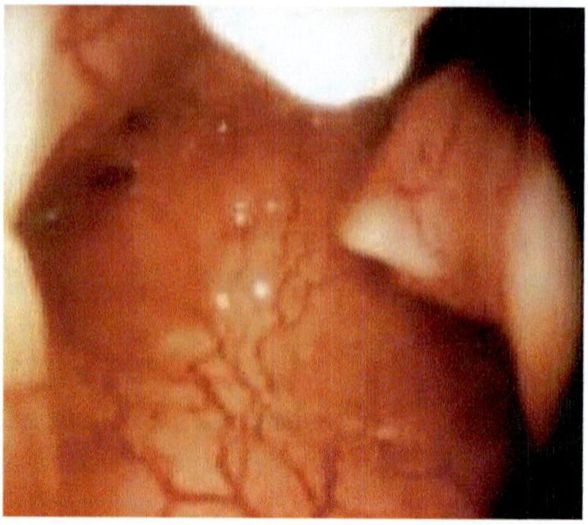

Fig. 17: Polypoid formation and increased vascularization.

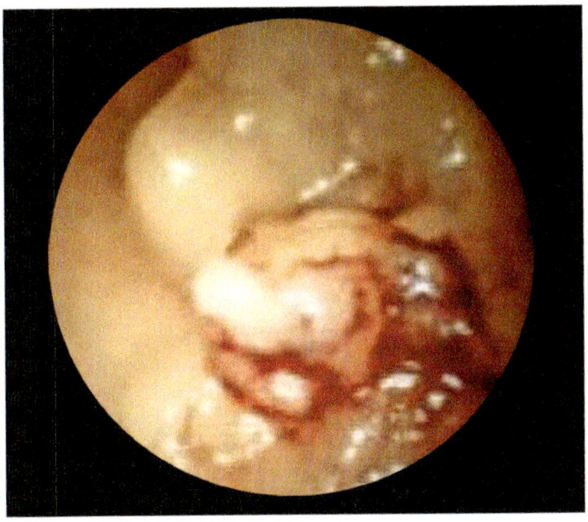

Fig. 18: Focal endometrial hyperplasia.

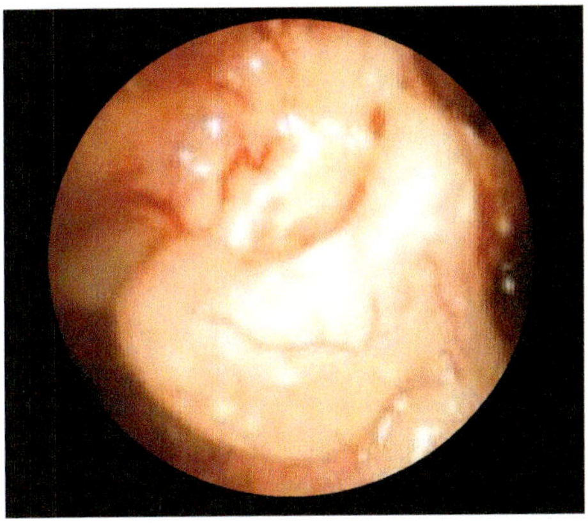

Fig. 19: Endometrial polypoid hyperplasia.

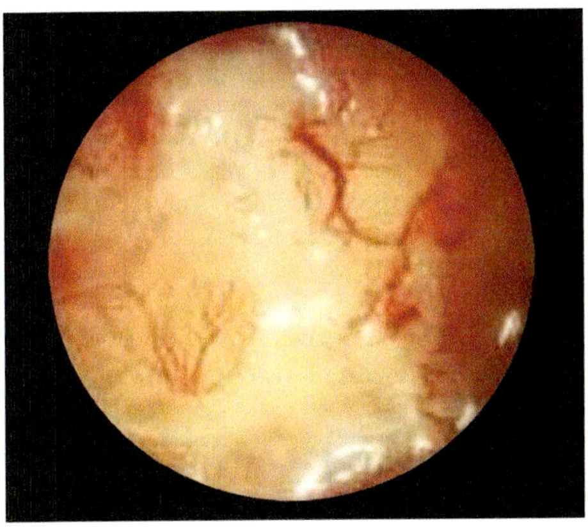

Fig. 20: High-risk endometrial hyperplasia, arborescent capillary vascularization.

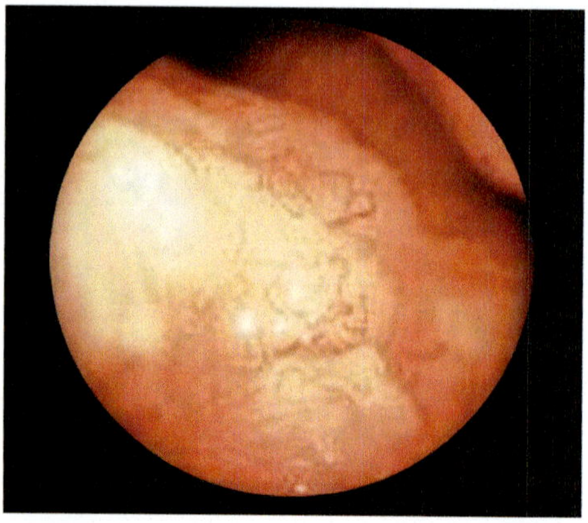

Fig. 21: High-risk endometrial corkscrew vascularization.

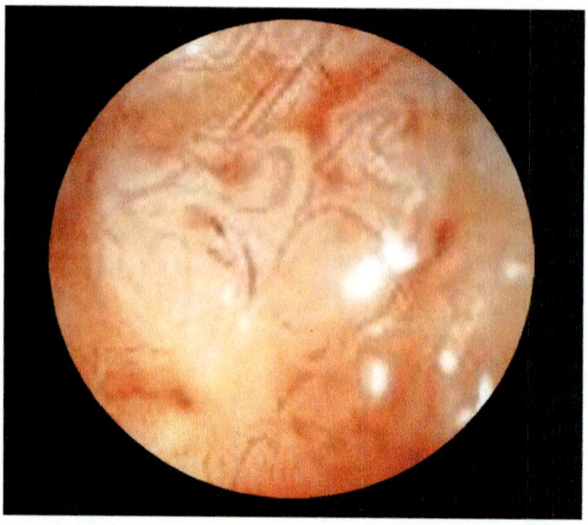

Fig. 22: Endometrial abnormal growth and abnormal vascularization.

Endometrial Intraepithelial Neoplasia: Hysteroscopic Aspects

The diagnosis of endometrial intraepithelial neoplasia (EIN) is best confirmed with hysteroscopy and endometrial biopsy. The hysteroscopic appearance of EIN is distinctive, characterized by an irregular, multilobulated surface with necrotic or spontaneously bleeding areas. The vascularization of these lesions is disorganized and irregular **(Figs. 23 to 27)**. Focal neoplastic lesions, often located near the tubal cornual areas, may be missed during blind curettage or endometrial aspiration **(Figs. 28 to 30)**. Hysteroscopy allows these focal lesions to be visualized and biopsied accurately.[11,12]

Hysteroscopy in Screening for Endometrial Carcinoma

Hysteroscopy is considered the gold standard for investigating AUB, especially in cases where endometrial carcinoma is suspected. Although hysteroscopy

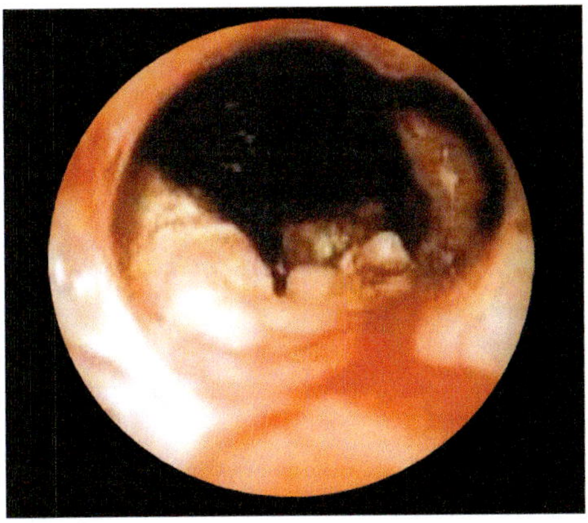

Fig. 23: Endometrial cancer, view from the isthmus.

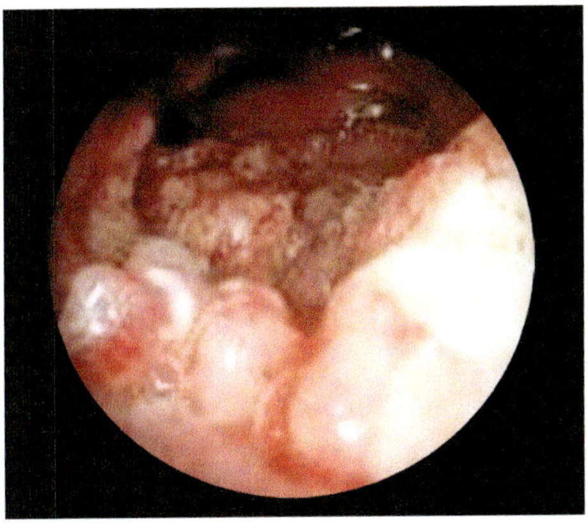

Fig. 24: Endometrial cancer, view of the uterine cavity.

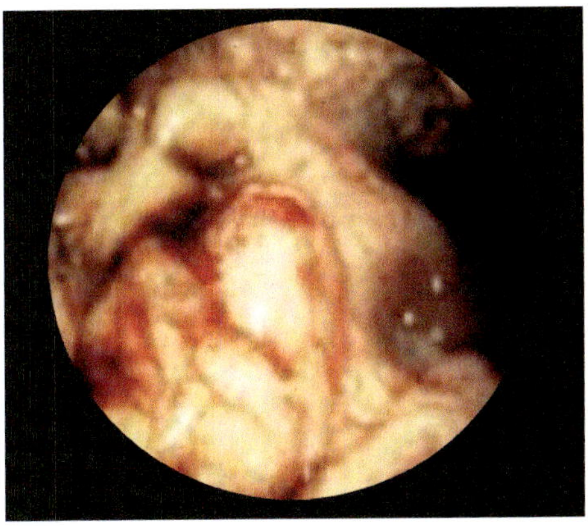

Fig. 25: Endometrial cancer polypoid and necrotic aspect.

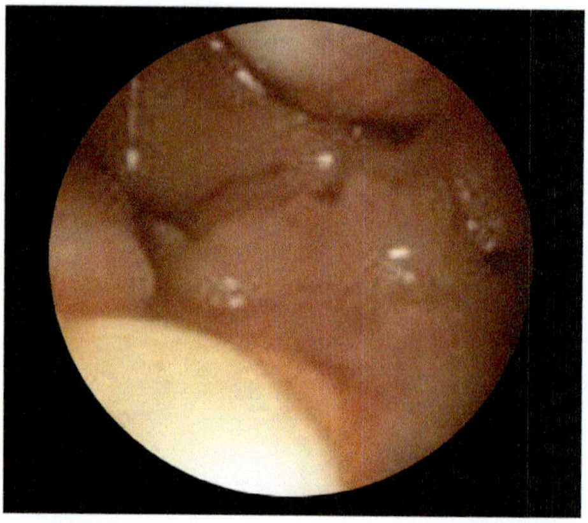

Fig. 26: Endometrial cancer, well-differentiated form.

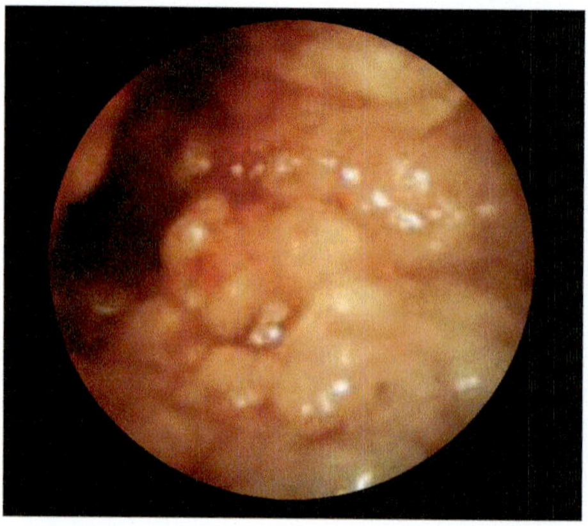

Fig. 27: Endometrial cancer invading the uterine cavity.

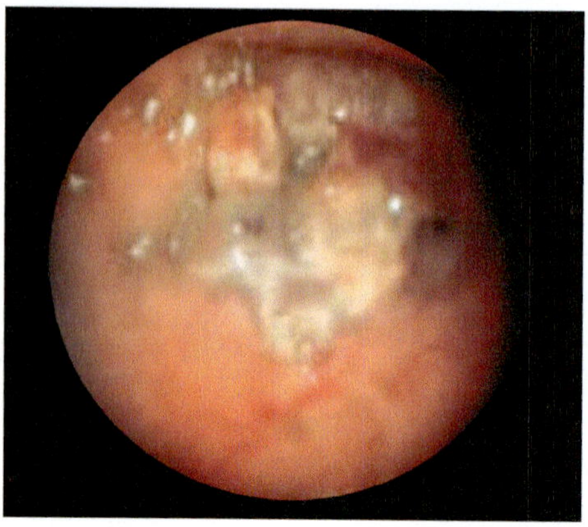

Fig. 28: Endometrial cancer—focal localization.

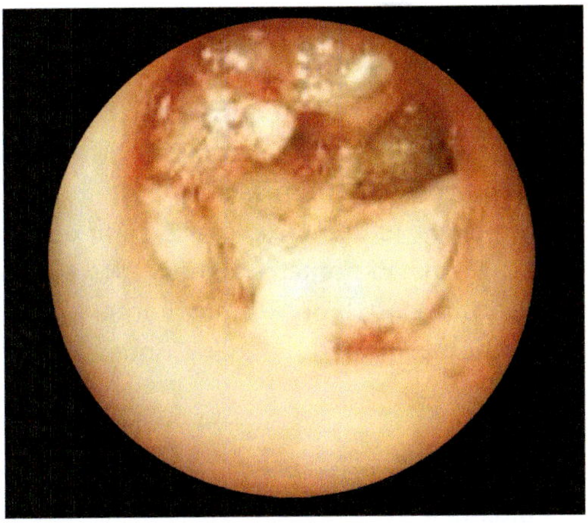

Fig. 29: Endometrial cancer of fundal localization.

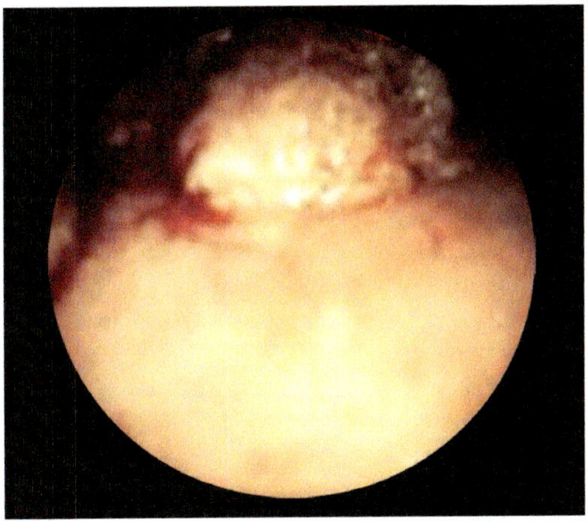

Fig. 30: Endometrial cancer with clearly circumscribed boundary between normal and neoplastic epithelium.

offers high diagnostic accuracy for endometrial carcinoma, it should not be the sole diagnostic tool. It should be used in combination with an endometrial biopsy to confirm the diagnosis.[13] Hysteroscopy helps identify patients who may not require further investigation if no pathology is observed. However, the need for biopsy in the absence of pathology is determined by the surgeon's experience. With increasing experience, the distinction between benign and malignant lesions can be made with a 20% false-positive rate and no false negatives. Combining hysteroscopy with guided biopsy raises the diagnostic accuracy for malignancy to 100%.[6] Concerns regarding the potential spread of malignant cells during hysteroscopic irrigation of the endometrial cavity are debated, with no consensus on the issue.[14]

CONCLUSION

It is noteworthy that, in 40% of pre- and postmenopausal women with AUB, no intrauterine pathology is identified as the source of bleeding. Conversely, 60% of these women are diagnosed with pathologies such as submucous myomas, polyps, or hyperplasia via hysteroscopy. Among postmenopausal women, polyps, endometrial cancer, and endometrial atrophy are more commonly detected. Endometrial biopsy is essential for confirming hysteroscopic findings, although biopsies may not be necessary in cases of normal or atrophic endometrium, thus saving time and reducing costs for both patients and physicians.

REFERENCES

1. Kotdawala P, Kotdawala S, Nagar N. Evaluation of endometrium in perimenopausal abnormal uterine bleeding. J Midlife Health. 2013;4(1):16-21. doi: 10.4103/0976-7800.109628. PMID: 23833528; PMCID: PMC3702059.
2. Donnez J, Dolmans MM. Uterine fibroid management: from the present to the future. Hum Reprod Update. 2016;22(6):665-86. doi: 10.1093/humupd/dmw023. Epub 2016 Jul 27. PMID: 27466209; PMCID: PMC5853598.
3. Rosales-Ortiz S, Na Shieli Barrón Martínez T, Sulvaran Victoria D, Arias Alarcon J, Márquez-Acosta J, Fugarolas Marín J. Bleeding and hysteroscopy in uterine myomatosis [Internet]. Fibroids. IntechOpen; 2021. Available from: http://dx.doi.org/10.5772/intechopen.94174.
4. Ngo YG, Fu HC, Chu LC, Tseng CW, Chen CY, Lee CY, et al. Specific hysteroscopic findings can efficiently distinguish the differences between malignant and benign endometrial polyps. Taiwanese J Obstet Gynecol. 2020;59(1):85-90. doi: 10.1016/j.tjog.2019.11.013.
5. Hennuru R, Potnuru R. Abnormal uterine bleeding in women of perimenopausal age: a retrospective study. Int J Reprod Contracept Obstet Gynecol. 2019;8:2406-9.
6. Telang M, Tanvir T. Understanding the endometrium at menopause: a hysteroscopist's view. J Midlife Health. 2021;12(3):232-6. doi: 10.4103/jmh.jmh_152_21. Epub 2021 Oct 16. PMID: 34759706; PMCID: PMC8569464.
7. Guarino A, Di Benedetto L, Assorgi C, Rocca A, Caserta D. Conservative and timely treatment in retained products of conception: a case report of placenta accreta retention. Int J Clin Exp Pathol. 2015;8(10):13625-1. PMID: 26722586; PMCID: PMC4680531.
8. Foreste V, Gallo A, Manzi A, Riccardi C, Carugno J, Sardo ADS. Hysteroscopy and retained products of conception: an update. Gynecol Minim Invasive Ther. 2021;10(4):203-9. doi: 10.4103/GMIT.GMIT_125_20. PMID: 34909376; PMCID: PMC8613498.
9. Sebastian A, Neerudu SR, Rebekah G, Varghese L, Regi A, Thomas A, et al. Risk factors for endometrial carcinoma in women with postmenopausal bleeding. J Obstet Gynaecol India. 2021;71(4):417-23. doi: 10.1007/s13224-021-01464-3. Epub 2021 Mar 14. PMID: 34566302; PMCID: PMC8418577.
10. Nees LK, Heublein S, Steinmacher S, Juhasz-Böss I, Brucker S, Tempfer CB, et al. Endometrial hyperplasia as a risk factor of endometrial cancer. Arch Gynecol

Obstet. 2022;306(2):407-21. doi: 10.1007/s00404-021-06380-5. Epub 2022 Jan 10. PMID: 35001185; PMCID: PMC9349105.

11. Pace L, Actis S, Mancarella M, Novara L, Mariani L, Perrini G, et al. Clinical, Sonographic, and hysteroscopic features of endometrial carcinoma diagnosed after hysterectomy in patients with a preoperative diagnosis of atypical hyperplasia: a single-center retrospective study. Diagnostics. 2022;12(12):3029. doi: 10.3390/diagnostics12123029.
12. Vitale SG, Riemma G, Carugno J, Chiofalo B, Vilos GA, Cianci S, et al. Hysteroscopy in the management of endometrial hyperplasia and cancer in reproductive aged women: new developments and current perspectives. Transl Cancer Res. 2020;9(12):7767-77. doi: 10.21037/tcr-20- 2092. PMID: 35117379; PMCID: PMC8799018.
13. Garuti G, Angioni S, Mereu L, et al. Hysteroscopic view with targeted biopsy in the assessment of endometrial carcinoma. What is the rate of underestimated diagnosis? The results of a multicenter Italian trial. Gynecol Surg. 2020;17:10. doi: 10.1186/s10397-020-01077-0.
14. Du Y, Xu Y, Qin Z, Sun L, Chen Y, Han L, et al. The oncology safety of diagnostic hysteroscopy in early-stage endometrial cancer: a systematic review and meta-analysis. Front Oncol. 2021;11:742-61. doi: 10.3389/fonc.2021.742761. PMID: 34745963; PMCID: PMC8566916.

6 CHAPTER

Diagnostic Hysteroscopy

Anupama Bhute

OVERVIEW

Diagnostic hysteroscopy is a procedure performed for direct visualization of the endometrial cavity to evaluate various abnormalities, thus enabling to diagnose issues related to abnormal bleeding, infertility, and other intrauterine pathologies.[1] Hysteroscopy is considered gold-standard technique for assessment and treatment of intrauterine pathologies.

Broadly, diagnostic hysteroscopy is categorized into two types: Panoramic and contact hysteroscopy.

1. Panoramic hysteroscopy implies a procedure where a liquid or gaseous distention media is used to distend uterine cavity. This is the routine followed method of hysteroscopy.
2. Contact hysteroscopy contrarily is the procedure where distension media is not utilized and thus is a time-consuming procedure with more complications. This method is not followed routinely.

INDICATIONS

Diagnostic hysteroscopy is performed to evaluate vaginal walls, cervix, endocervical canal, endometrial cavity and tubal ostia[2] is indicated for several conditions, including:

- Abnormal uterine bleeding (AUB)
- Postmenopausal bleeding
- *Infertility and recurrent miscarriages:* To assess the uterine cavity for structural abnormalities like fibroids, polyps, or congenital malformations that might impair fertility or cause recurrent pregnancy loss.
- *Retained products of conception:* To locate and remove retained tissues after miscarriage or delivery.
- *Evaluation of uterine anomalies:* To diagnose and assess congenital uterine anomalies such as septate uterus.
- *Suspected intrauterine pathology:* Polyps, fibroids, adhesions, and hyperplasia or malignancy of the endometrium.
- Removal of foreign bodies like intrauterine contraceptive device (IUCD), retained fetal bones.
- Rule out endometrial cancer.[3]

CONTRAINDICATIONS

- *Absolute contraindications:* Active pelvic infection, prodromal or active genital herpes, and confirmed cervical or endometrial cancer[4]
- *Relative contraindications:* Moderate vaginal bleeding

EQUIPMENT

Two types of hysteroscopes are available—flexible and rigid. Hysteroscopes with angles from 0 to 70° range are available. These are easily connected to a light source, a video-monitoring system, and fluid channels. For the best possible visualization of the endometrial cavity, a constant flow of distending media is required. An operative channel on the majority of hysteroscopes allows surgical instruments like tiny hysteroscopic graspers, scissors, or a tenaculum to pass through.

DISTENSION MEDIA

For satisfactory hysteroscopy, suitable distention of the uterus is required. Liquid and gaseous distension media are widely used. However, gaseous distension media like carbon dioxide is only used during diagnostic hysteroscopies since visibility is mislaid with bleeding.[5] Liquid distension media allows better irrigation of the cavity for improved picturing. Distension media essentially should be carefully chosen, whenever performing operative hysteroscopy and using thermal loops. Liquids containing electrolytes must not be used with monopolar current since there is risk of energy diffusion to surrounding tissues. While using bipolar instruments, electrolyte-rich liquid-distending media, such as normal saline, may be carefully chosen.[6]

Timing of Procedure

Women in postmenopausal age group can undergo hysteroscopy at any point of time. In case of premenopausal women, procedure is avoided during the secretory phase of menstrual cycle as endometrium may appear polypoidal and there are chances of misdiagnosis.

Premedications

- Preprocedure antibiotics are not required.[7]
- Currently, there are no recommendations for giving analgesics on routine basis.
- Misoprostol is not recommended on a routine basis, however is being used by many practitioners.[8]

Anesthesia

Diagnostic hysteroscopy performed on an outpatient basis is generally does not require any anesthesia, some procedures are carried out under local anesthesia.

Diagnostic hysteroscopy is performed in an outpatient clinic where equipment to handle cardiac emergencies are available.

PROCEDURE

The procedure typically follows these steps:

- A written informed consent is taken prior to initiation of procedure.
- The patient is positioned in the lithotomy position, with a flat table and avoiding Trendelenburg position. A bimanual pelvic examination should be carried out to evaluate vagina, cervix, size of uterus, mobility of uterus. The hysteroscope is assembled, the camera is white-balanced and focused, and the inflow tract is optimized.
- *Vaginoscopy technique:* Vaginoscopy in initiated by introducing the hysteroscope into the vagina. The vagina is then expanded, and the cervix and external os are visualized by lightly advancing the scope. The posterior fornix is usually easily identified. Once the external os is located, the hysteroscope is cautiously introduced and passed into the uterine cavity.
- *Traditional technique:* A speculum is first inserted, cervix is visualized and grasped anteriorly with a single-tooth tenaculum, cervix is then dilated to the diameter of the hysteroscope being used, hysteroscope is inserted. At the same time, counter traction is applied with the tenaculum to straighten the uterus. Uterine cavity may be evaluated for any pathology and a plan made for the operative interference. The bilateral tubal ostia should be recognized at the commencement of the procedure.

Documentation

Findings are documented, and if necessary, biopsies are taken for further pathological evaluation.

RISKS AND COMPLICATIONS

Although generally safe, diagnostic hysteroscopy carries potential risks, including:

- Uterine perforation and cervical lacerations can occur in 0.6–1% of procedures.[9] Patients are monitored and if hemodynamically stable are manages conservatively.
- *Fluid overload:* Although common in operative hysteroscopies (operative hysteroscopy intravascular absorption or OHIA) can rarely occur in diagnostic hysteroscopies. This complication can be avoided by optimizing amount of fluid being used for distention as per a recent recommendations by the British Society of Gynaecological Endoscopy (BSGE) and European Society of Gynaecological Endoscopy (ESGE) on fluid management where upper threshold for isotonic media is 2500 mL and for hypotonic fluids is 1000 mL in healthy women.[5]

- Infection
- Embolism is common in cases where carbon dioxide is used as distention media.[10] Immediate resuscitation, Durant's position (left lateral decubitus and Trendelenburg position) abandoning procedure are essential in management.
- Adverse drug reactions to anesthetic drugs

CONCLUSION

Diagnostic hysteroscopy is a valuable tool in modern gynecology, providing direct insight into the uterine cavity and aiding in the diagnosis of various intrauterine conditions. Targeted sampling and full resection of uterine abnormalities like polyps are possible with hysteroscopy and direct visualization of the entire uterine cavity, as opposed to blind endometrial sampling. Continuous advancements in technology and techniques promise to further enhance its diagnostic and therapeutic capabilities.

REFERENCES

1. Salazar CA, Isaacson KB. Office Operative Hysteroscopy: An Update. J Minim Invasive Gynecol. 2018;25(2):199-208.
2. Ignaszak-Kaus N, Chmaj-Wierzchowska K, Nowak A, Wszołek K, Wilczak M. An overview of outpatient hysteroscopy. Clin Exp Obstet Gynecol. 2022;49(8):181.
3. Du Y, Xu Y, Qin Z, Sun L, Chen Y, Han L, et al. The Oncology Safety of Diagnostic Hysteroscopy in Early-Stage Endometrial Cancer: A Systematic Review and Meta-Analysis. Front Oncol [Internet]. 2021 Oct 21 [cited 2024 Jul 19];11. Available from: https://www.frontiersin.org/journals/oncology/articles/10.3389/fonc.2021.742761/full.
4. Moore JF, Carugno J. Hysteroscopy. In: StatPearls [Internet]. Treasure Island (FL): StatPearls Publishing; 2024 [cited 2024 Jul 30]. Available from: http://www.ncbi.nlm.nih.gov/books/NBK564345/.
5. Umranikar S, Clark TJ, Saridogan E, Miligkos D, Arambage K, Torbe E, et al. BSGE/ESGE guideline on management of fluid distension media in operative hysteroscopy. Gynecol Surg. 2016;13(4):289-303.
6. Abdallah KS, Gadalla MA, Breijer MC, Mol BWJ. Uterine distension media for outpatient hysteroscopy. Cochrane Database Syst Rev. 2021;2021(11):CD006604.
7. ACOG Practice Bulletin No. 195: Prevention of infection after gynecologic procedures. Obstet Gynecol. 2018;131(6):e172-89.
8. Hua Y, Zhang W, Hu X, Yang A, Zhu X. The use of misoprostol for cervical priming prior to hysteroscopy: a systematic review and analysis. Drug Des Devel Ther. 2016;10:2789-801.
9. Aas-Eng MK, Langebrekke A, Hudelist G. Complications in operative hysteroscopy: is prevention possible? Acta Obstet Gynecol Scand. 2017;96(12):1399-403.
10. Verma A, Singh MP. Venous gas embolism in operative hysteroscopy: a devastating complication in a relatively simple surgery. J Anaesthesiol Clin Pharmacol. 2018;34(1):103-6.

7

CHAPTER

Fertility Enhancing Hysteroscopy

Nilesh Balkawade, Sharayu Bhagat

INTRODUCTION

Hysteroscopy is a minimally invasive procedure that allows direct visualization of the uterine cavity using a hysteroscope. In infertility evaluations, various pathologies that might impair infertility can be diagnosed and treated.[1]

WHY IS HYSTEROSCOPY IMPORTANT?

Hysteroscopy is considered the gold standard for visualization of the uterine cavity, and it helps in simultaneous detection and treatment of intracavitary anomalies with greater accuracy than other methods. Due to improved endoscopic developments, can be performed reliably and safely as an office procedure. The most common uterine abnormalities, including endometrial polyps, submucosal myomas, uterine septum and intrauterine adhesions, are common in infertile women. It is object of debate whether diagnostic and/or operative hysteroscopy should be considered in the basic workup of infertile couple.[2]

TYPES OF HYSTEROSCOPY (FLOWCHART 1 AND TABLE 1)

Flowchart 1: Types of hysteroscopy.

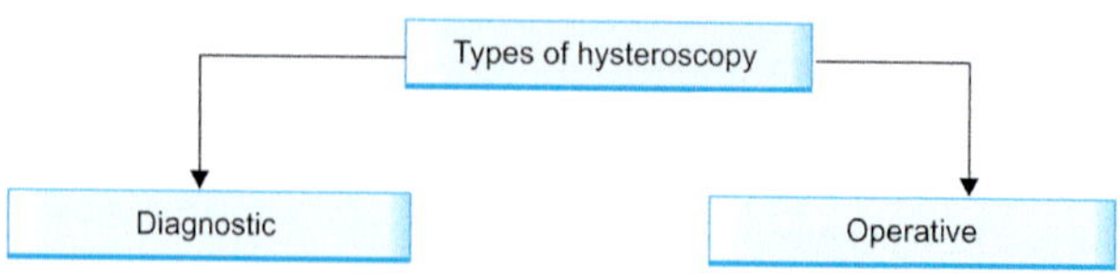

TABLE 1: Types of hysteroscopy.

• Inspection of uterine cavity for any abnormalities • Office hysteroscopy—done with minimal discomfort • It is often used to confirm abnormal findings found in saline sonohysterography or 3D ultrasound	• Used to treat conditions such as polyps, submucous fibroids, or adhesions (Asherman's syndrome). Identified during diagnostic hysteroscopy • It is performed under anesthesia in a hospital setting • Surgical instruments can be passed through the hysteroscope for corrective measures

INDICATIONS FOR HYSTEROSCOPY IN INFERTILITY

Unexplained infertility: When initial fertility workup shows no apparent cause.

Recurrent implantation failure: Recurrent implantation failure (RIF) is often related to underlying uterine abnormalities. After multiple failed in vitro fertilization (IVF) attempts, hysteroscopy helps ensure the uterine cavity is optimal for embryo transfer.

In TROPHY Trial (2016)—702 women with normal TVS and 2–4 unsuccessful IVF cycles, hysteroscopy showed no difference in livebirth rate, implantation rate and miscarriage rate.

Recurrent pregnancy loss: Recurrent pregnancy loss (RPL), often defined as two or more consecutive miscarriages. Uterine factors such as adhesions, polyps, or congenital malformations like a septate uterus are common causes of RPL, which contribute to miscarriage. Hysteroscopically diagnosed major intrauterine abnormalities in 7% of women with recurrent abortions and allows for precise diagnosis and treatment.[3]

Uterine cavity abnormalities: Suspected from other diagnostic tools such as ultrasound or hysterosalpingography (HSG).

Endometrial polyps: Can distort the endometrial cavity, reducing the chances of implantation.

Submucous fibroids: These fibroids, particularly when they encroach into the uterine cavity, can negatively affect implantation and embryo development.

Intrauterine adhesions (Asherman's syndrome): Adhesions can cause partial or complete obstruction of the uterine cavity, preventing embryo implantation or leading to miscarriage.

CONTRAINDICATIONS

- Acute pelvic inflammatory disease (PID)
- Active herpes infection
- Pregnancy
- Medically unstable patient **(Fig. 1)**

ROLE OF HYSTEROSCOPY IN IVF (TABLE 2)

TABLE 2: Pre- and post-IVF evaluation in hysteroscopy.

Pre-IVF evaluation	*Post-failed IVF cycles*
Many fertility specialists recommend hysteroscopy as a part of the routine evaluation before IVF to ensure there are no intrauterine pathologies that could compromise implantation[4]	• In patients with multiple failed IVF cycles, hysteroscopy can be used to assess any potential uterine issues that might have been missed in earlier evaluations • *Endometrial scratching:* During hysteroscopy, endometrial scratching can be performed to stimulate a favorable environment for embryo implantation in subsequent IVF cycles[5]

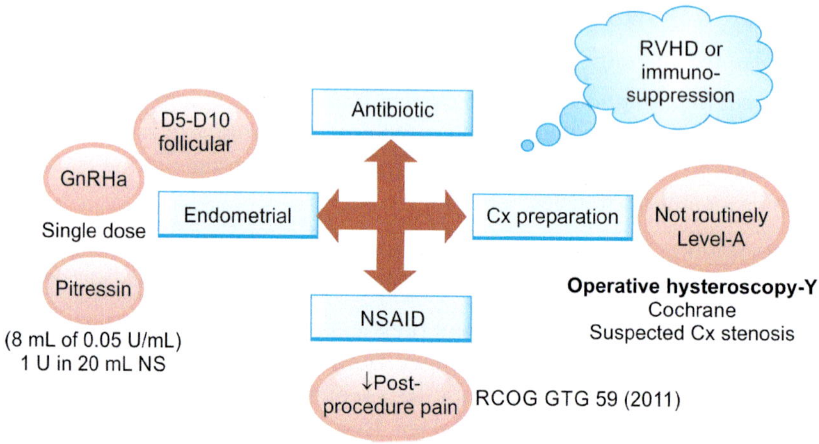

Fig. 1: Preoperation preparation.

TECHNIQUES USED IN ART (TABLE 3)

TABLE 3: Techniques in ART.

Office hysteroscopy	*Operative hysteroscopy*
• It is done as an OPD procedure and does not require general anesthesia • Mostly used for diagnostic purpose • Minimal discomfort to the patient • Polyps, small fibroids, or adhesions can be identified • Miniature hysteroscopes (2.7 mm with a 3–3.5 mm sheath) should be used for diagnostic outpatient hysteroscopy as they significantly reduce the discomfort experienced by the woman. (Level A)—RCOG	• It is performed under general anesthesia in a surgical setting • It is used as diagnostic and operative procedures • Instruments passed through the hysteroscope are used to correct the abnormalities • This procedure is used to treat conditions such as fibroids, polyps, adhesions, or congenital anomalies

ROLE OF HYSTEROSCOPY IN DIAGNOSING UTERINE PATHOLOGIES

Endometrial Polyps

Endometrial polyps represent one of the mostly can be asymptomatic. They are benign growths that can interfere with implantation and affect fertility. Studies have shown that hysteroscopic removal of polyps significantly improves IVF outcomes by restoring normal uterine anatomy and enhancing endometrial receptivity. Yanaihara et al. found the highest pregnancy rate (57%) after hysteroscopic excision of polyp located in the uterotubal junction, which could cause loss of function of the ostium and affect sperm passage.[6] The available low-quality evidence suggests that the

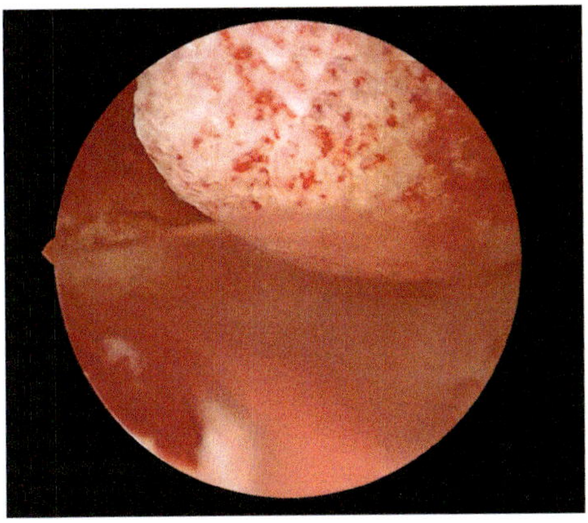

Fig. 2: Endometrial polyps.

hysteroscopic removal of endometrial polyps suspected on ultrasound in women prior to IUI may improve the clinical pregnancy rate compared to simple diagnostic hysteroscopy[7] **(Fig. 2)**.

Submucosal Myoma

The incidence of submucosal myomas associated with infertility is estimated between 5 and 10%.[8] Myoma that protrude into the uterine cavity (submucous fibroids) are associated with reduced implantation rates and increased miscarriage risk. According to retrospective and case control studies, the presence of myomas that protrude into the endometrial cavity decreases pregnancy and implantation rates in patients seeking spontaneous pregnancy or planning to undergo IVF. Fertility rate after hysteroscopic myomectomy should increase, especially for large myomas. A Cochrane systematic review has shown that SIS and hysteroscopy to be equivalent for the diagnosis of submucous leiomyomas, with both superior to transvaginal ultrasonography (TVUS)[9] **(Fig. 3)**.

Chronic Endometritis

Hysteroscope helps to diagnose micropolyps, stromal edema, strawberry App which are suggestive of chronic endometritis **(Fig. 4)**.

Isthmocele

'Double Arch' is a diagnostic sign typically seen with isthmocele in hysteroscopy. It allows for direct visualization of the defect **(Figs. 5A and B)**.

Intrauterine Adhesions (Asherman Syndrome)

Intrauterine adhesions are associated with infertility and recurrent pregnancy failure. Adhesions form within the uterine cavity, often as a

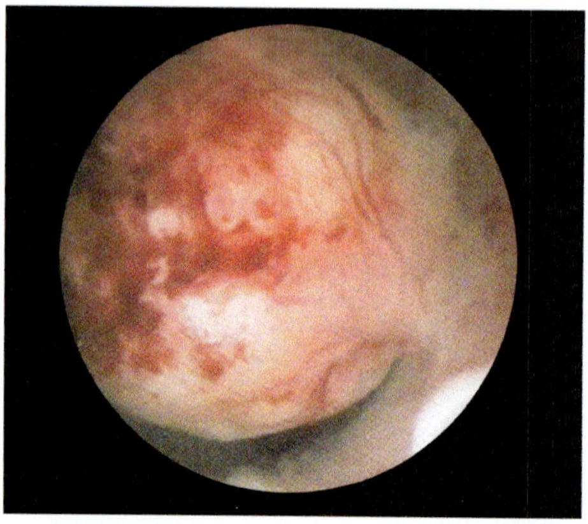

Fig. 3: Submucosal myoma.

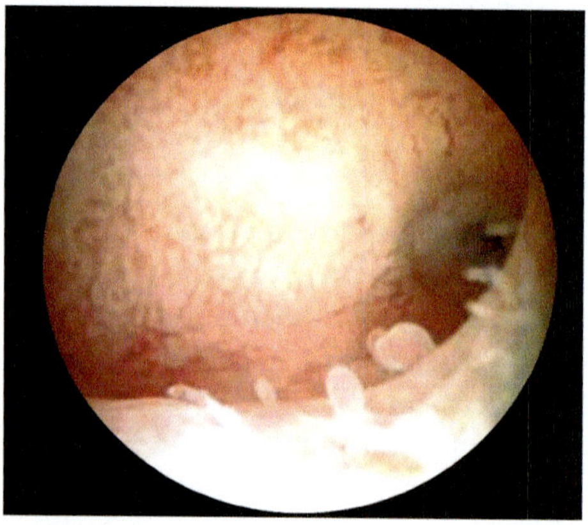

Fig. 4: Chronic endometritis.

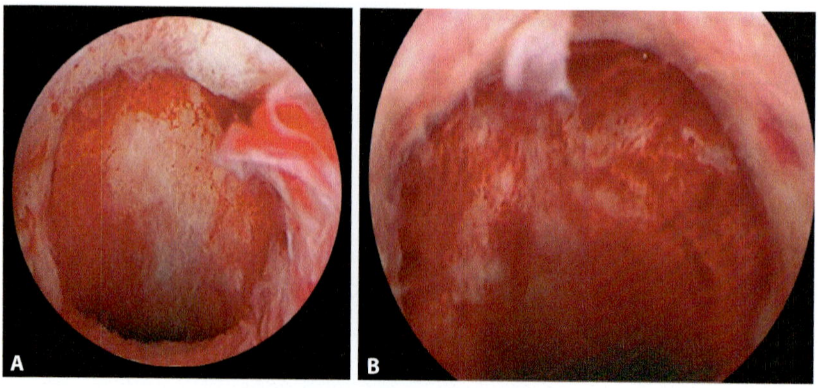

Figs. 5A and B: Isthmocele.

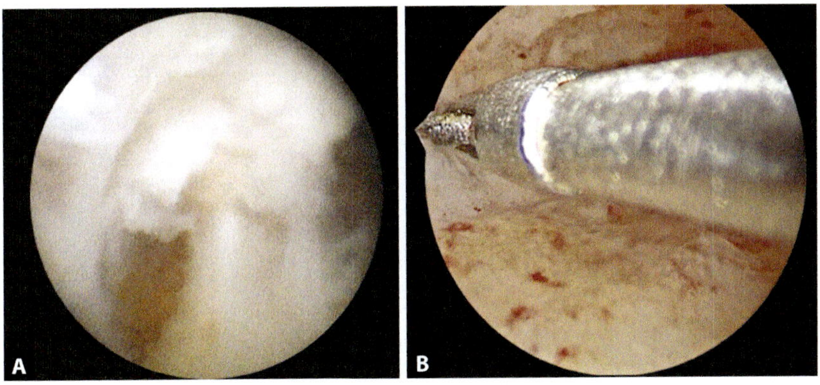

Figs. 6A and B: Asherman syndrome.

result of previous surgeries, infections, or trauma, leading to infertility and miscarriage. Hysteroscopic adhesiolysis is a well-established procedure to restore normal uterine architecture and function **(Figs. 6A and B)**.

Congenital Uterine Anomalies

- 4% of infertile women, and 10–15% of patients with recurrent miscarriage have Müllerian anomalies.[10]
- Congenital uterine anomalies are caused by defects in development or fusion of the Müllerian ducts. The uterus septum is the most frequent uterine malformation (0.2–2.3%) of reproductive age women, and it is associated with the highest risk of infertility, pregnancy loss, preterm birth and fetal malpresentation.
- Uterine malformations had a 53% viable pregnancy rate compared with 89% normal uteri.
- Poor viability rates more with:
    - Unicornuate (12–62%)
    - T-shaped (18–49%)
    - Didelphic (32–52%)
    - Septate (26–94%) uteri[11]

> It is recommended that imaging with hysteroscopy should be used to diagnose uterine septa rather than laparoscopy with hysteroscopy because this approach is less invasive (Grade B)—ESHRE/ASRM.

Hysteroscopic septum resection is the current standard procedure to restore the normal uterine cavity to improve pregnancy outcome congenital uterine anomalies, such as a septate uterus, are linked to infertility and recurrent pregnancy loss. Hysteroscopic resection of the septum is a minimally invasive procedure that improves reproductive outcomes by normalizing the uterine cavity.

ASRM recommends hysteroscopic resection	ESHRE, NICE, and RCOG do not support the routine used of the procedure

ASRM, 2016 guidelines:

- In a patient with infertility, prior pregnancy loss, or poor obstetrical outcome it is reasonable to consider septum incision **(Fig. 7)**. (Grade C)
- In a patient without infertility or prior pregnancy loss, it may be reasonable to consider septum incision following counseling regarding potential risks and benefits of the procedure **(Fig. 8)**. (Grade C)

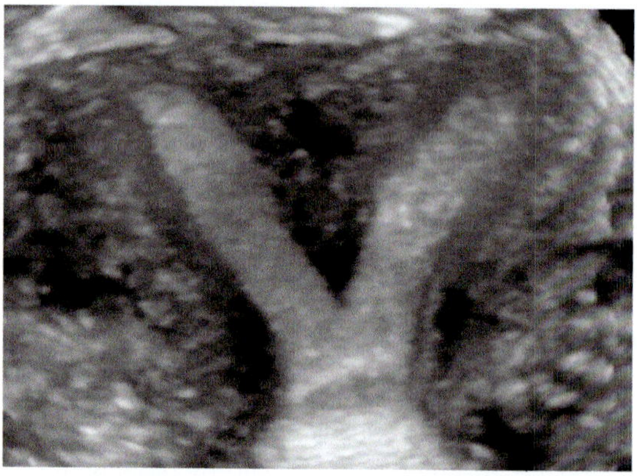

Fig. 7: Patient with infertility, prior pregnancy loss, or poor obstetrical outcome, it is reasonable to consider septum incision.

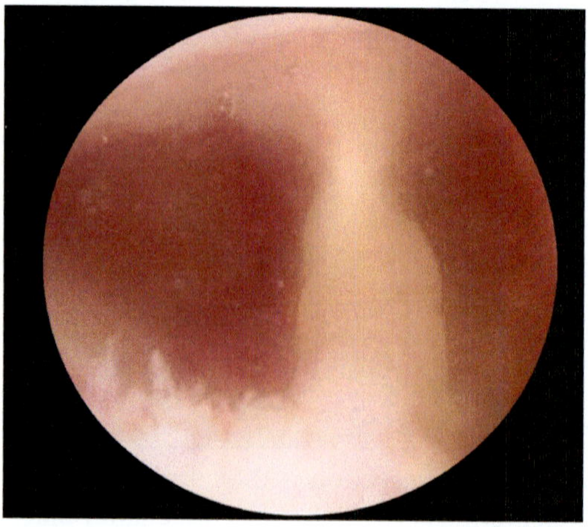

Fig. 8: Patient without infertility or prior pregnancy loss, it may be reasonable to consider septum incision following counseling regarding potential risks and benefits of the procedure.

RECENT EVIDENCE ON THE IMPACT OF HYSTEROSCOPY ON IVF OUTCOMES

Recent research highlights the benefits of hysteroscopy in improving IVF outcomes, especially for women with RIF or RPL. A meta-analysis concluded that women who underwent hysteroscopy prior to IVF had higher implantation and livebirth rates compared to those who did not.[12] Similarly, a study showed that hysteroscopic polypectomy improved pregnancy rates in women undergoing IVF, suggesting that even small polyps can have a significant impact on implantation.[13]

Other studies suggest that hysteroscopy may enhance endometrial receptivity by inducing a mild inflammatory response in the endometrium, which may improve implantation rates in subsequent IVF cycles. In a study, the authors hypothesized that endometrial injury caused by hysteroscopy may increase the expression of cytokines and adhesion molecules, thus promoting embryo implantation.[14]

RISKS AND LIMITATIONS

Infection: Postoperative infection is rare but possible, and prophylactic antibiotics may be administered to reduce this risk.

Uterine perforation: When a hysteroscope punctures the uterine wall. It is more common in operative hysteroscopies and may require additional surgical intervention.

Adhesion formation: In some cases, operative hysteroscopy can lead to the formation of new adhesions, particularly in women with a history of intrauterine adhesions (Asherman syndrome).

Bleeding: Minimal bleeding is common following hysteroscopy, but significant hemorrhage is rare and may require intervention.

Anesthesia-related complication: Despite these risks, hysteroscopy is widely considered a safe and effective procedure with a low complication rate.

CONCLUSION

Recent advancements have made hysteroscopy safer, faster, and more effective. Hysteroscopy is a valuable tool in the evaluation and treatment of infertility, especially in uterine abnormalities. It enhances the diagnosis and management of intrauterine conditions that could hinder implantation or cause recurrent pregnancy loss. Hysteroscopy can significantly improve the chances of a successful pregnancy.

REFERENCES

1. Moore JF, Carugno J. Hysteroscopy [Internet]. StatPearls. Treasure Island (FL): StatPearls Publishing; 2023 [updated 2023 Jul 18; cited 2024 Oct 3].
2. Gulisano M, Gulino FA, Incognito GG, Cimino M, Dilisi V, Di Stefano A, et al. Role of hysteroscopy on infertility: The eternal dilemma. Clin Exp Obstet Gynecol. 2023;50(5):99.
3. Genovese F, Di Guardo F, Monteleone MM, D'Urso V, Colaleo FM, Leanza V, Palumbo M. Hysteroscopy as an investigational operative procedure in primary and secondary infertility: a systematic review. Int J Fertil Steril. 2021;15(2):80-7.
4. Zikopoulos A, Galani A, Siristatidis C, Georgiou I, Mastora E, Paraskevaidi M, et al. Is hysteroscopy prior to IVF associated with an increased probability of live births in patients with normal transvaginal scan findings after their first failed IVF trial? J Clin Med. 2022;11(5):1217.
5. Van Hoogenhuijze NE, Kasius JC, Broekmans FJM, Bosteels J, Torrance HL. Endometrial scratching prior to IVF; does it help and for whom? A systematic review and meta-analysis. Hum Reprod Open. 2019;2019(1):hoy025.
6. Yanaihara A, Yorimitsu T, Motoyama H, Iwasaki S, Kawamura T. Location of endometrial polyp and pregnancy rate in infertility patients. Fertil Steril. 2008;90:180-2.
7. Van Wessel S, Weyers S, Broekmans FJ, D'Hooghe TM, Bongers MY, Mol BWJ, et al. Hysteroscopy for treating subfertility associated with suspected major uterine cavity abnormalities. Cochrane Database Syst Rev;2018.
8. Guo XC, Segars JH. The impact and management of fibroids for fertility: an evidence-based approach. Obstet Gynecol Clin North Am. 2012;39(4):521-33. doi: 10.1016/j.ogc.2012.09.005. PMCID: PMC3608270. PMID: 23182558.
9. Rezk A, Kahn J, Singh M. Fertility sparing management in uterine fibroids [Internet]. StatPearls. Treasure Island (FL): StatPearls Publishing; 2023 [updated 2023 Jun 7; cited 2024 Oct 3].
10. Chan YY, Jayaprakasan K, Zamora J, Thornton JG, Raine-Fenning N, Coomarasamy A. The prevalence of congenital uterine anomalies in unselected and high-risk populations: a systematic review. Hum Reprod Update. 2011;17(6):761-71. doi: 10.1093/humupd/dmr028. PMCID: PMC3191936. PMID: 21705770.
11. Hosseinirad H, Yadegari P, Mohanazadeh Falahieh F, Keivanlou Shahrestanaki J, Karimi B, Afsharzadeh N, Sadeghi Y. The impact of congenital uterine abnormalities on pregnancy and fertility: a literature review. JBRA Assist Reprod. 2021;25(4):608-16. doi: 10.5935/1518-0557.20210021. PMCID: PMC8489822. PMID: 34224238.
12. Mao X, Wu L, Chen Q, Kuang Y, Zhang S. Effect of hysteroscopy before starting in-vitro fertilization for women with recurrent implantation failure: a meta-analysis and systematic review. Medicine (Baltimore). 2019;98(7): e14075.
13. Al Chami A, Saridogan E. Endometrial polyps and subfertility. J Obstet Gynaecol India. 2017;67(1):9-14. doi: 10.1007/s13224-016-0929-4. PMCID: PMC5306103. PMID: 28242961.
14. Papanikolaou E, Peitsidis N, Tsakiridis I, Michos G, Skalias A, Patoulias D, et al. Endometrial scratching during hysteroscopy in women undergoing in vitro fertilization: a systematic review and meta-analysis. Front Surg. 2023;10:1225111.

8

CHAPTER

Hysteroscopic Myomectomy

Rohan Palshetkar, Mayuri More, Chiranjeev Shetty

INTRODUCTION

Fibroblasts and the smooth muscle of the myometrium are the source of uterine leiomyomas. Fibroids are the most prevalent tumors identified in the reproductive organs. Family history, alcohol consumption, obesity, soybean product intake, hypertension, red meat consumption, and vitamin D insufficiency have been linked to a higher prevalence of uterine fibroids.[1,2]

For the treatment of all women with abnormal uterine bleeding, infertility, and suspected intrauterine illness, direct visualization of the uterine cavity during hysteroscopy is essential for both diagnostic and therapeutic purposes. This minimally invasive method for the conservative treatment of intrauterine pathology has been made possible by technological advancements in optics, scope diameters, fluid management, tissue removal systems (TRS), and electrosurgery. This has made outpatient hysteroscopy more feasible and made many blind procedures less beneficial.

DIAGNOSIS[3]

Submucous myoma in the uterine cavity can be detected, counted, located, and correlated with the myometrium using accurate methods—Hysterosalpingography and hysteroscopy. Hysterosonography and pelvic ultrasonography, and transvaginal, and pelvic MRI offer a view of the uterus chamber and wall.[4]

Hysterosalpingography is beneficial for infertile patients as it includes tubal patency as well as configuration examination. It indicates myoma's existence, although its position on the myometrium is inefficient.[5]

Hysteroscopy which directly visualizes the uterine cavity, and provides complete information regarding the intracavitary submucous myoma and a favorable assessment of the intramural portion.

Ultrasonography (USG) transvaginal ultrasonography (TVUS), in particular, is the initial examination and is low-cost, easily accessible, and accurate;

nevertheless, posterior acoustic shadowing makes it challenging to assess and count many nodules and big uteruses. It is operator-dependent, but it aids in evaluating the intramural myoma and frees the myometrial mantle up to the serosa **(Fig. 1)**.

Hysterosonography: When distinguishing the uterine cavity and myometrial mantle, an ultrasound with the uterus dilated and saline solution for contrast and detailing is more accurate than a TVUS **(Fig. 2)**.

A pelvic MRI is recommended if the uterus contains more than four fibroids or a volume more than 375 cm^3.[2] Because of its exceptional

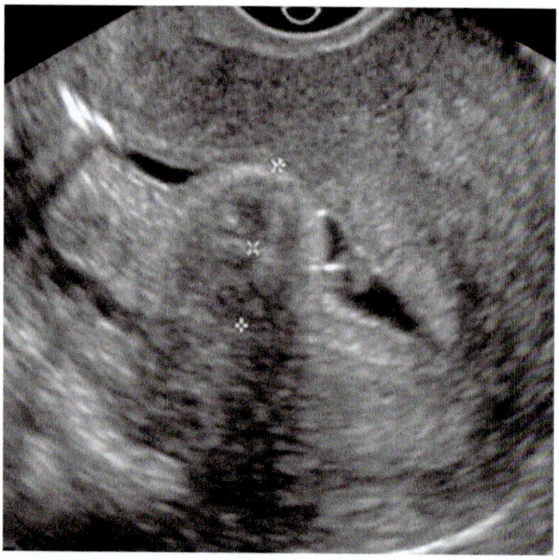

Fig. 1: Submucous myoma on ultrasound. (*Submucosal fibroid)

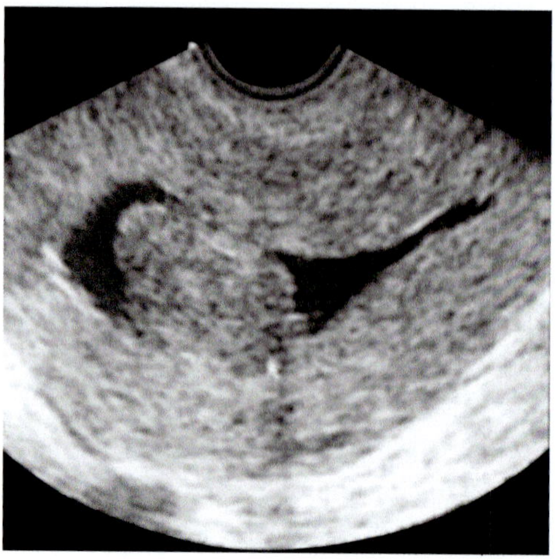

Fig. 2: Submucous myoma in sonohysterography.

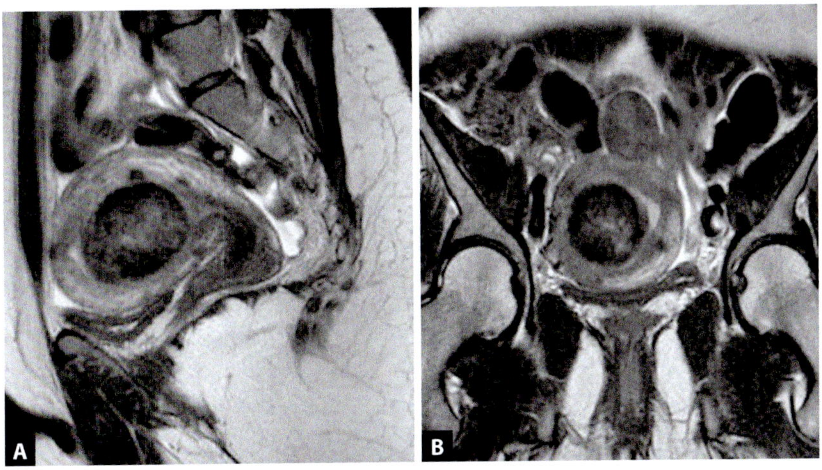

Figs. 3A and B: MRI with submucous myoma.

characterization of nodule number, position, size, and proximity, it is used to diagnose adenomyosis and adenomyoma, rule out nonfibroid sarcomas, and measure the myometrial mantle **(Figs. 3A and B)**.

Office hysteroscopy: Office hysteroscopy for diagnostic and therapeutic purposes has been made simpler by the introduction of smaller diameter scopes, flexible hysteroscopes, micro resectoscopes, and tissue removal technologies. This aids surgical planning and patient education.

CLASSIFICATION

The categorization of submucous myomas into standardized levels facilitates the assessment of the difficulty and complexity associated with hysteroscopic myomectomy, as well as the comparison of outcomes. As of right now, there are two main classifications: the Lasmar—STEP-W, which was published in 2005, and the ESGE, which was developed by Wansteker et al. in 1993 **(Tables 1 and 2)**.[6]

HYSTEROSCOPIC MYOMECTOMY TECHNIQUES

We have two strategies that can be combined or separated, and each has their own merits. Enucleation and slicing or myolysis may be done in inpatient and outpatient hysteroscopy.[7] Lasmar and Mazzon described enucleation in 2001 and 1995, respectively. A "cold loop" is used by Mazzon to break the nodule until it reaches the intramural part and mobilizes the fibroid, whereas Lasmar enucleates and cuts the fibroid completely. To access the pseudocapsule (Lasmar), cut the endometrium around the submucosal myoma or slice it near the myometrium (Mazzon).[8] Sectioning fibrous beams at the pseudocapsule is necessary. Because it does not sever myometrial

TABLE 1: ESGE submucous myoma classification—Wamsteker (1993).

Type	*Myoma portions inside of the cavity*
0	Totally inside
1	>50% inside
2	<50% inside

TABLE 2: Lasmar submucous myoma classification—STEPW classification (2005).

	Size	*Penetration*	*Base*	*Topography*	*Lateral wall*
0	≤2 cm	0	≤1/3	Lower	
1	>2–5 cm	≤50%	>1/3–2/3	Middle	+1
2	>5 cm	>50%	>2/3	Upper	
Score		+	+	+	
Score	*Group*	*Suggested treatment*			
0 to 4	I	Low complexity hysteroscopic myomectomy			
5 to 6	II	Complex hysteroscopic myomectomy, consider preparing with GnRH analog and/or 2-step surgery			
7 to 9	III	Recommend an alternative non-hysteroscopic technique			

Source: Lasmar RB et al., Minim Invasive Gynecol. 2005;12(4):308-11.

veins, mobilizing the myoma from the outside to the center and front to the rear releases it from the myometrium without causing bleeding, heat damage, or intravasation. All devices can mobilize and enucleate the myoma without energy, however, scissors or tweezers are better in outpatient clinics and Collins loop or "cold loop" in hospital hysteroscopy. The best method for hysteroscopic myomectomy is enucleation, which mobilizes the nodule and separates it from the uterine wall, whereas fragmentation eliminates the myoma from the uterine cavity.[9]

Slicing Technique

The slicing approach involves the incremental and systematic excision of the myoma in segments, commencing at its surface and progressively advancing toward its base. Slices of myoma are removed energetically from the fundus to the cervix using the semicircular loop in a mono- or bipolar resectoscope. Depending on the energy type, different distension media are used. For example, bipolar energy uses electrolytic media like 0.9% physiological saline and Ringer's lactate, while monopolar energy uses nonelectrolytic media like 1.5% glycine, mannitol, and mannitol/sorbitol.

Due to the accumulation of myoma fragments in the uterine cavity, it is essential to halt the treatment and evacuate the cavity to restore visibility of both the cavity and the myoma.

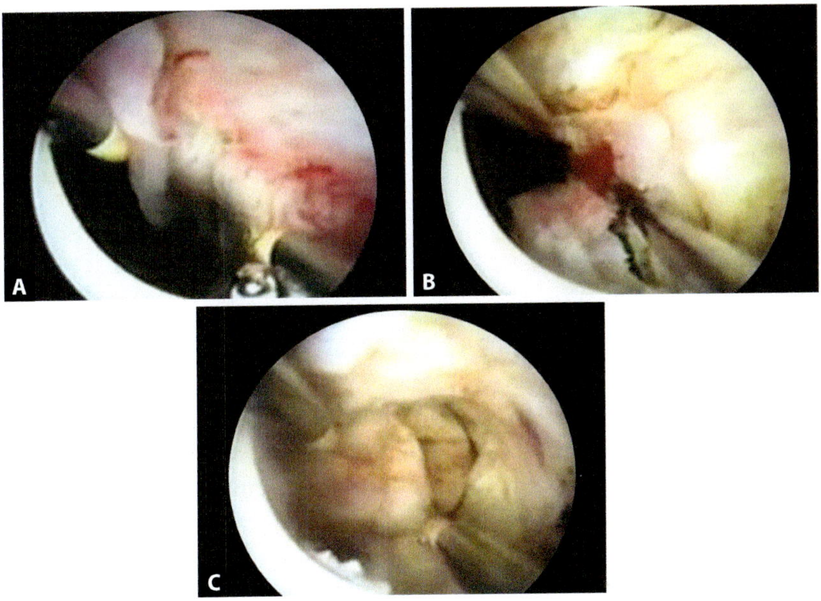

Figs. 4A to C: Slicing technique.

This method allows for the surgical treatment of bigger nodules, excision of myoma pieces from the cavity, simultaneous hemostasis, and volumetric reduction. The procedure presents several disadvantages, including increased bleeding due to the superficial nature of myoma vessels, a heightened risk of intravasation—particularly in myomas with substantial intramural components—an elevated likelihood of perforation, frequent surgical interruptions to excise fragments, and significant damage to the adjacent endometrial and myometrial tissues surrounding the myoma.

The speed of the loop's movement influences the balance between cutting and coagulation; a rapidly moving loop favors cutting over coagulation, whereas a slower loop enhances coagulation relative to cutting **(Figs. 4A to C)**.

Morcellation Technique

Hysteroscopic TRS executes the fragmentation and aspiration of endometrial abnormalities, including fibroids and polyps. Three primary brands are presently available in the market: Myosure, Truclear, and Symphion, which are predominantly utilized for kids 0 and 1 intrauterine leiomyomas. A swiftly moving blade excises tiny segments of the fibroid, which are subsequently aspirated into a tissue trap for pathological assessment. From the cavity, this approach eliminates the necessity for the extraction of fibroid "chips".

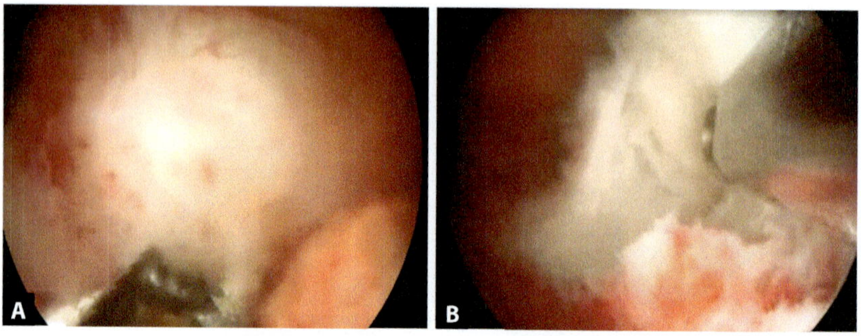

Figs. 5A and B: Morcellator technique—hysteroscopic mechanical tissue removal.

Hysteroscopic TRS has presented an effective and user-friendly instrument for hysteroscopic myomectomy. Morcellators have seen increased utilization and acceptability, particularly among novice hysteroscopic surgeons, owing to their ease of use, brief learning curve, and reliance solely on mechanical rather than energy-based methods, demonstrating effective outcomes in the management of intracavitary lesions. The boundaries encompass primarily intramural lesions, as well as lesions located in the cornual and fundic regions **(Figs. 5A and B)**.

Laser Technique

The application of Laser will cause myolysis, which will either result in the myoma's destruction or a delayed expulsion after ischemia and volume decrease. Consequently, it may be applicable for nodules with a significant intramural component, when resectoscope surgery could entail hazards. The predominant LASER utilized in hysteroscopy is the diode laser apparatus, featuring a 5 Fr fiber, proficient in combining 2 distinct wavelengths: 980 m and 1470 nm. Hemoglobin absorbs wavelengths of 980 nm more easily, which improves coagulation action.

When using Laser fiber for enucleation, the endometrium is cut until the pseudocapsule is reached. The nodule is then either mechanically mobilized with a second instrument or allowed to expel spontaneously. If an intracavitary myoma is present, a second hysteroscopy with a resectoscope is scheduled for one to two months later (the OPPIuM Technique) **(Figs. 6A to C)**.

Radiofrequency Ablation Technique

This is an additional ultrasound-guided myolysis technique. This method uses a radiofrequency ablation handpiece connected to an intrauterine ultrasound probe to form a single device that allows the rods to pass through the myoma. With the use of this real-time ultrasound integration, the physician may see and target several fibroids for therapy.

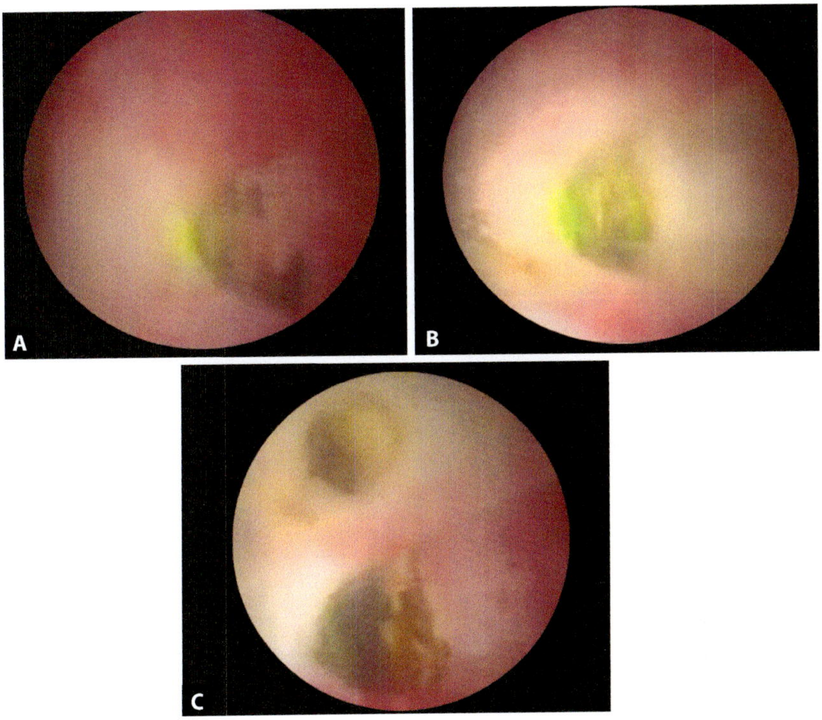

Figs. 6A to C: Laser in submucous myoma with deep intramural component.

Mazzon's Cold Loop Technique

Mazzon's 1995 approach involves resecting the submucosal myoma with a semicircle loop resectoscope and mono- or bipolar energy until the intramural portion is reached. After reaching the pseudocapsule, the loop becomes stiffer and unenergized (cold loop), mechanically mobilizing the myoma till enucleation. After leaving the myoma free in the uterine cavity, an energy loop fragments and removes it. The myometrium can be approached without current, reducing the danger of perforation and thermal harm to adjacent organs, hemorrhage, and intravasation **(Figs. 7A to F)**.

Mobilization and Enucleation Technique Using the Pssedocapsule—Lasmar

The 2002 Lasmar approach is called "direct mobilization of the myoma". The Collins loop resectoscope is used to incise the endometrium around the myoma in the submucosa to release fibrous beams at the pseudocapsule. After identifying the pseudocapsule with the same device, the myoma is separated from the myometrium and slides into it like in laparotomic

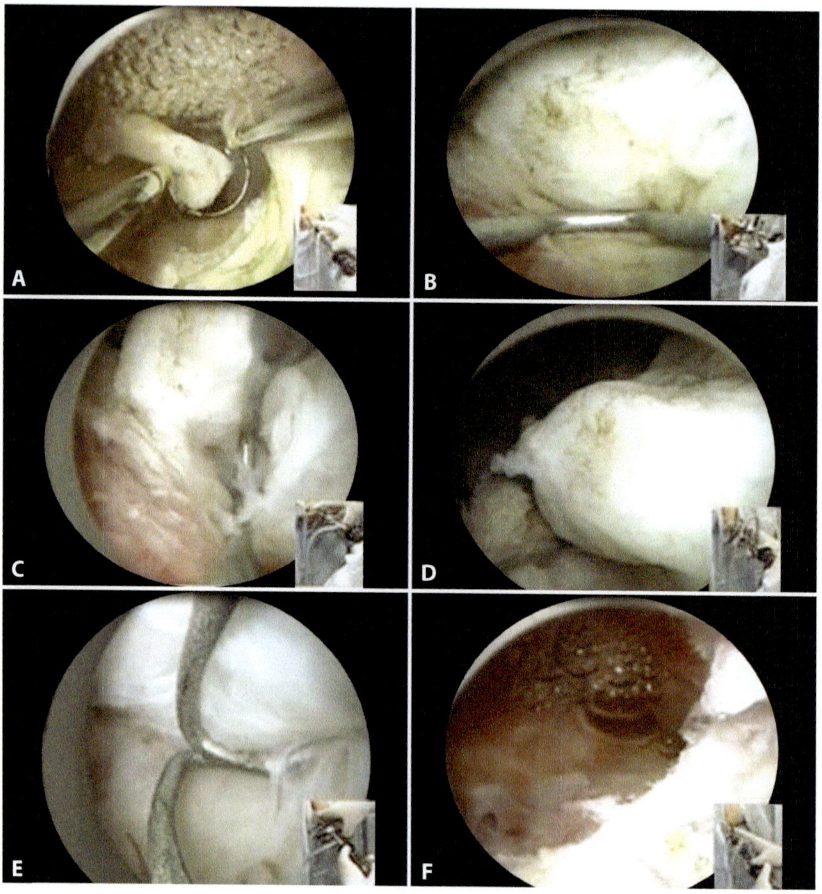

Figs. 7A to F: Mazzon's cold loop technique.

and laparoscopic myomectomy. By moving the Collins loop with the hysteroscope from the lateral to the central area of the myoma, parallel to the nodule, the myoma migrates into the uterine cavity until it is fully liberated. When the myometrium, which has been squeezed by the nodule, returns to its normal position, the pseudocapsule relaxes, causing the intramural lesion to become intracavitary. Like all myoma enucleation methods, this one reduces perforation, heat damage to the myometrium, hemorrhage, as well as intravasation. With the myoma completely or almost completely in the cavity, the Collins loop slices the nodule longitudinally to remove it in large pieces, boosting efficiency. This method increases the limit of hysteroscopic myomectomy from 10 to 3 mm depending on the myometrial mantle measurement before surgery **(Figs. 8A to F)**.

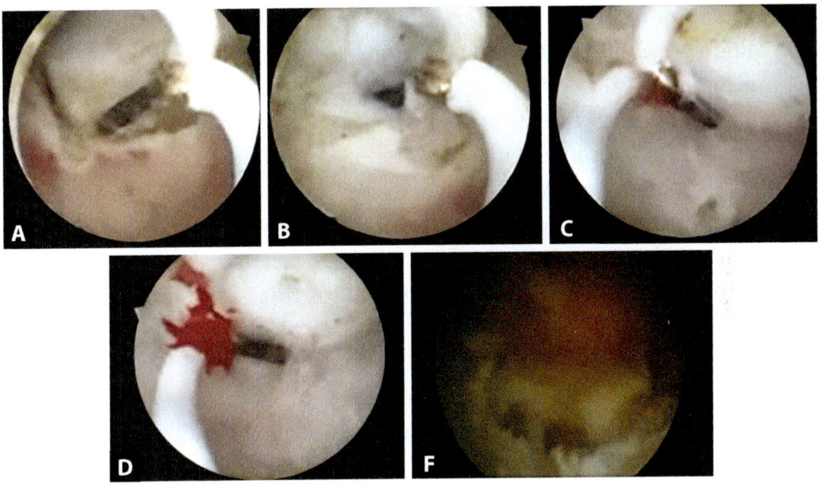

Figs. 8A to F: OR hysteroscopic myomectomy, with Collins electrode, enucleation, and preserving pseudocapsule.

COMPLICATIONS

Myomectomy has the most complications of all hysteroscopic operations. Hysteroscopic myomectomy complication rate is 0.8–2.6%.[10,11]

- *Cervical laceration:* The forceps and Hegar dilators can cause cervix laceration during dilation, especially in older patients and those who used GnRH before the surgery. Tamponade and/or suturing the laceration site works well.
- *Uterine perforation:* this can happen following surgery or cervical dilatation. Surgery is rarely required when it happens without energy; instead, a few hours of hospitalization and clinical monitoring are sufficient. The procedure must be terminated since uterine distention is not achievable, and the patient will return for surgery in three months. Investigation of the pelvic and abdominal cavities is required if energy was used during perforation, regardless of the outcome. Injuries in bowel and bladder can be ruled out by laparoscopy or laparotomy. For fluid balance complex myomectomy, patients have bladder catheterization, so hematuria may indicate bladder damage. Hematuria only happens when the uterine front wall ruptures, though it can also happen subtly when a bladder catheter is replaced. Cystoscopy should be done prior to laparoscopy. Without laparoscopy/laparotomy, intestinal injury is harder to suspect, especially heat injuries that can take 3 days to fistulize and cause peritonitis and sepsis. Vascular lesions may cause hemodynamic instability.
- *Uterine bleeding:* Myomas' superficial vessels or myometrial bed might cause uterine hemorrhage. Vascular coagulation, antihemorrhagic drugs,

oxytocin, and an intracavitary Foley's catheter with a well-distended balloon are administered for 4–12 hours. While the patient is observed, as was previously described.

- *Fluid overload:* Limit fluid balance to 1000 mL negative and avoid 2000 mL. Pulmonary edema, heart failure, encephalopathy, brain injury, convulsions, coma, and death can result from rapid and substantial fluid consumption. Massive absorption of 1.5% glycine produces nausea, vomiting, and disorientation. Excess intravascular fluid can result in encephalopathy, brain injury, hyponatremia, ammonia, overload, hemodilution, and even death. Complication severity is strongly related to volume absorbed quickly. Longer surgeries can increase distention medium absorption. Electrolyte problems can be avoided by bipolar current and saline and ringer lactate, but not fluid excess or heart failure.
- *Infections:* Residues and the internal os occlusion can cause hematometrium and pyometra in myomectomy, but hysteroscopic operations seldom cause infection.
- *Air embolism* is a rare yet deadly condition. Ambient air may enter the venous circulation via cervical canal dilation or by a myometrium continuity solution, with greater risk in the Trendelenburg position, where the uterus and heart are situated. Hysteroscopic myomectomy and other hysteroscopic surgeries have similar air embolism risks.
- *Late problems:* Like adhesions and placenta accreta can occur after major resections. Some publications report 1–13% adhesions following hysteroscopic myomectomy.[12]

CLINICAL OUTCOMES

- *Abnormal uterine bleeding (AUB):* It has been reported that 70–99% of hysteroscopic myomectomy procedures are successful. The success rate is influenced by the size, quantity, and the fibroids' position, as well as the proficiency of the surgeon and the completeness of the resection.[13]
- *Reproductive outcomes:* Submucosal fibroids are often associated with subfertility, as well as hysteroscopic myomectomy is typically advised; nevertheless, the existing evidence is inconsistent on this matter. The American Society for Reproductive Medicine's (ASRM) Practice Committee developed guidelines outlining the connection between leiomyomas and fertility. Formulating exact results that can guide practice recommendations is made more difficult by the variety of study populations, types, locations, quantities, and sizes of fibroids, as well as the inclusion and exclusion criteria.[14]

CONCLUSION

The most difficult and involved hysteroscopic procedure—with the highest risks and potential complications—is hysteroscopic myomectomy. It is the most effective treatment option for submucous myomas and is safe and effective for managing intrauterine problems.

There are two distinct phases in which the safety of myomectomy is evaluated: preoperative assessment and the actual surgical surgery. Preoperative care includes uterine fibroids classification, recognizing the patient's desire for future pregnancy, and hemodynamic assessment.

REFERENCES

1. Stewart, EA. Uterine fibroids. The Lancet. 2015;379 (9816):2342-51. https://doi.org/10.1016/S0140-6736(12)60044-0.
2. Khan AT, Shehmar M, Gupta JK. Uterine fibroids: Current perspectives. International Journal of Women's Health. 2014;6:95-114. https://doi.org/10.2147/IJWH.S51083].
3. Hirst A, Dutton S, Wu O, Briggs A, Edwards CA. A multicentre retrospective cohort study comparing methods for the diagnosis of uterine fibroids. British Medical Journal. 2016;355:i5847. https://doi.org/10.1136/bmj.i5847.
4. Dueholm M, Lundorf E, Hansen ES, Sorensen JS, Ledertoug S. Accuracy of magnetic resonance imaging and transvaginal ultrasonography for the diagnosis of adenomyosis. Human Reproduction. 2001;16(11):2418-22. https://doi.org/10.1093/humrep/16.11.2418.
5. Lasmar RB, Barrozo PR, Dias R, Oliveira MA. Submucous myomas: a new presurgical classification to evaluate the viability of hysteroscopic surgical treatment—preliminary report. J Minim Invasive Gynecol. 2005;12(4):308-11. https://doi.org/10.1016/j.jmig.2005.04.021.
6. Wamsteker K, Emanuel MH, De Kruif JH. Transcervical hysteroscopic myomectomy: A classification to predict the complexity and outcome of the procedure. BJOG. 1993;100(8):679-82. https://doi.org/10.1111/j.1471-0528.1993.tb14226.x.
7. Mazzon I. (1995). Hysteroscopic myomectomy: A comprehensive review of the literature. Surgical Technology International. 1995;4: 140-6. https://pubmed.ncbi.nlm.nih.gov/7553038/.
8. Lasmar RB, Barrozo PR. Hysteroscopic myomectomy in the treatment of submucous myomas. Journal of Minimally Invasive Gynecology. 2002;9(1):52-6. https://doi.org/10.1016/S1553-4650(02)00056-1.
9. Emanuel MH, Wamsteker K. Hysteroscopic myomectomy: Techniques and strategies to improve outcomes. Reproductive BioMedicine Online. 2005;11(4):478-83. https://doi.org/10.1016/S1472-6483(10)61220-7.
10. Litta P, Saccardi C, Conte L, Fabris A. Hysteroscopic myomectomy: techniques and complications. Minerva Ginecologica. 2010;62(1):1-6. https://pubmed.ncbi.nlm.nih.gov/20083945/.
11. Lasmar RB, Lasmar BP, Moawad NS. Hysteroscopic Myomectomy. Medicina. 2022;58(11):1627. https://doi.org/10.3390/medicina58111627.

12. Donnez J, Jadoul P. Hysteroscopic myomectomy and pregnancy outcomes. Fertility and Sterility. 2002;79(3):456-60. https://doi.org/10.1016/S0015-0282(02)02942-7.
13. Pritts EA, Parker WH, Olive DL. Fibroids and infertility: an updated systematic review of the evidence. Fertility and Sterility. 2009;91(4):1215-23. https://doi.org/10.1016/j.fertnstert.2008.01.051.
14. Bosteels J, Kasius JC, Weyers S, Broekmans FJ, Mol BWJ, D'Hooghe, TM. Hysteroscopy for treating subfertility associated with suspected major uterine cavity abnormalities. Cochrane Database of Systematic Reviews. 2015;2:CD009461. https://doi.org/10.1002/14651858.CD009461.pub3.

9 CHAPTER

Asherman's Management

Neharika Malhotra, Narendra Malhotra

INTRODUCTION

Asherman's syndrome refers to the formation of adhesions and/or fibrosis within the uterine cavity. It is also known by other terms such as 'intrauterine adhesions,' uterine synechiae, sclerotic endometrium, endometrial sclerosis, or Fritsch-Asherman syndrome. The condition was initially described by Heinrich Fritsch in 1894 and later classified by Joseph Asherman in 1948. It affects 5–39% of women with recurrent pregnancy loss.

The syndrome typically occurs due to trauma to the basal layer of the endometrium, often following surgical procedures like dilatation and curettage, cesarean section, myomectomy, or as a result of chronic endometritis from pelvic inflammatory disease, including genital tuberculosis. Key symptoms include secondary amenorrhea, hypomenorrhea, and infertility. Hysteroscopy is considered the gold standard for diagnosis, as it allows for direct evaluation of the extent of scar tissue formation.

Intrauterine adhesions leading to amenorrhea following curettage were first reported by Fritsch in 1894. Later, in 1950, Asherman detailed the cases of 29 women who developed amenorrhea as a result of trauma to the uterine cavity, now recognized as Asherman's syndrome (AS). AS is characterized by the presence of adhesions within the uterus or endocervix, resulting in risks such as hypomenorrhea or amenorrhea, reduced fertility, pregnancy loss, and abnormal placentation.

RISK FACTORS

Trauma caused by surgical interventions, primarily curettage of the basal layer of the endometrium shortly after a pregnancy, is the main reason for development of symptomatic IUA. These adhesions can result in partial or complete obstruction of the uterine cavity or the cervical canal. An incidence of 10% IUA after one curettage evaluated by HSG was seen in one randomized controlled trial. However, in women with at least two curettages 30.6% (22/72) had IUA when evaluated by hysteroscopy 10 weeks after the curettages.

STAGING

Most of the patients had history of primary or secondary infertility 15% of patients were nullipara with history of surgical trauma or any infection process causing intrauterine scarring Dr Warnsteker Staging, which was used (methods for staging, was done by sonohysterography and by 3D ultrasonography).

Stage I: <25% of the cervical canal and cavity affected **(Fig. 1)**.

Stage II: <50% of cervical canal and cavity affected **(Fig. 2)**.

Stage III: <75% of the cervical canal and cavity affected **(Fig. 3)**.

Stage IV: More than 75% of cervical canal and cavity affected. The surgical technique for treatment consists of resection of scar tissue using hysteroscopic microinstruments **(Fig. 4)**.

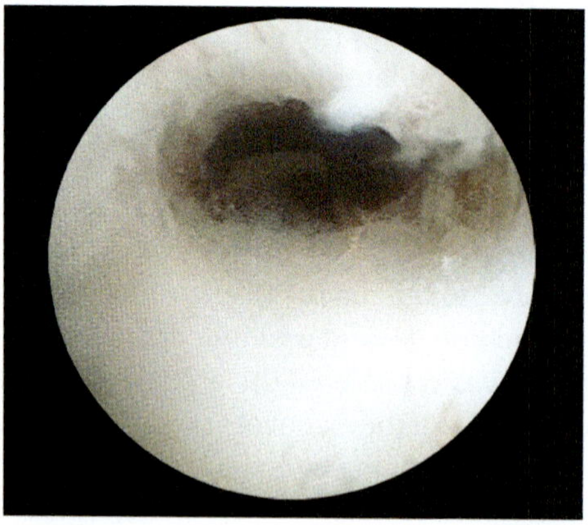

Fig. 1: The cervical canal and cavity affected less than 25% (Stage I).

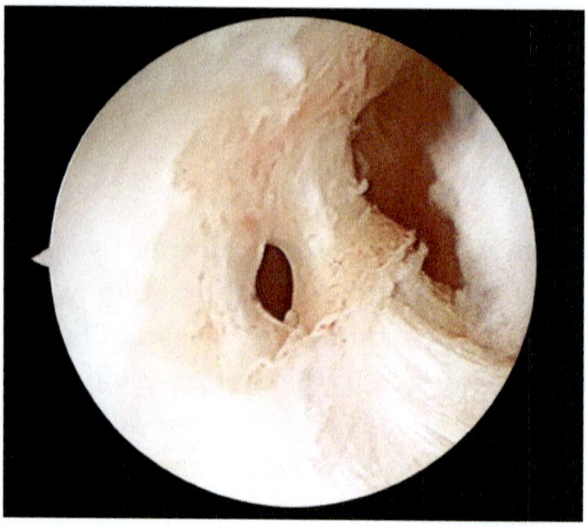

Fig. 2: The cervical canal and cavity affected less than 50% (Stage II).

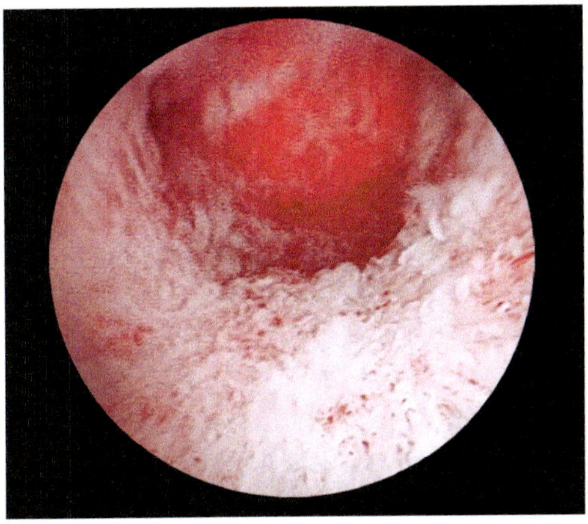

Fig. 3: The cervical canal and cavity affected less than 75% (Stage III).

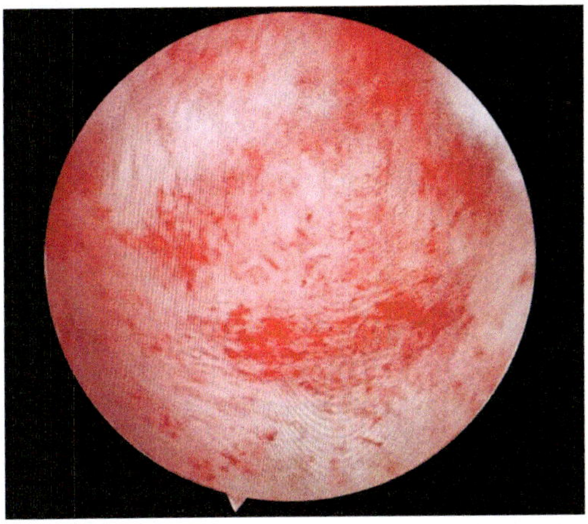

Fig. 4: The cervical canal and cavity affected more than 75% (Stage IV).

TREATMENT

Hysteroscopic adhesiolysis is the primary treatment for intrauterine adhesions, with postoperative care varying based on the severity of the condition. The different hysteroscopic methods used for adhesiolysis are outlined below:

Plain Hysteroscopy

Simple distension of the uterine cavity combined with blunt adhesiolysis using the hysteroscope itself can effectively treat delicate adhesions. Additionally, blunt dissection with a resectoscope and a Collins knife may be used for adhesion removal.

Monopolar Current

A resectoscope, along with glycine as the distension medium, is used to cut and coagulate tissue through the application of monopolar current.

Bipolar Current

Bipolar electrosurgery is employed to cut and coagulate adhesions and scar tissue, using isotonic distension media such as VersaPoint.

Scissors

This is the safest modality used which mechanically cuts the adhesions. This is the mainstay in our method of management practice. This cuts the adhesions and also prevents any further collateral damage, which might occur due to using of any electrical or energy source to do so. Also complications that occur due to perforations in this surgery when using scissors remain simple and not complex and hence are easier to manage.

Laser

Nd:YAG laser energy is delivered by fiber inserted through operating hysteroscope, which leads to vaporization of the tissue up to the depth of 5–6 mm.

Photo showing Grade 2 Asherman's with cavity compromised with adhesions **(Fig. 5)**.

Photo showing normalized cavity with adhesions having been removed **(Fig. 6)**.

Photo showing hysteroscopic resection of the adhesion with scissor **(Fig. 7)**.

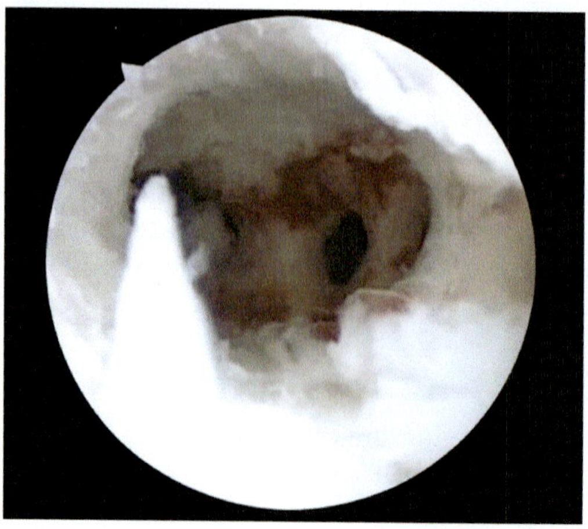

Fig. 5: Grade 2 Asherman's with cavity compromised with adhesions.

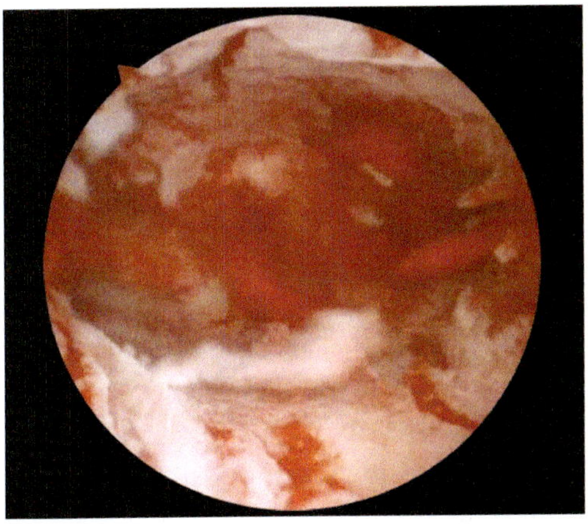

Fig. 6: Normalized cavity with adhesions having been removed.

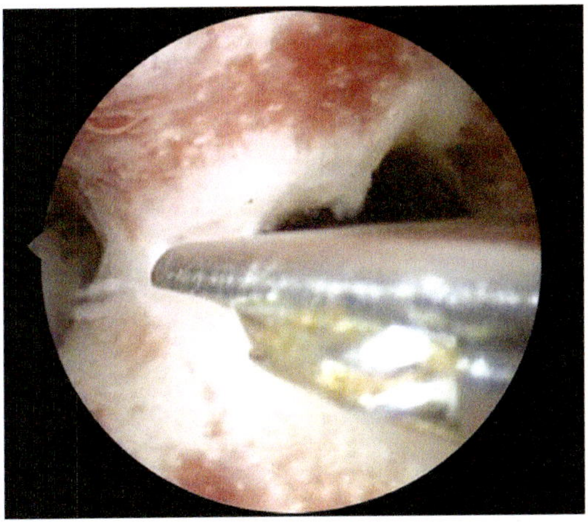

Fig. 7: Hysteroscopic resection of the adhesion with scissor.

POSTOPERATIVE PROTOCOL

Mild

High doses of conjugated equine estrogen (up to 4–5 mg daily) for 21 days followed by medroxyprogesterone 20 mg daily is given and a relook hysteroscopy is done after next period.

Moderate and Severe

An inert intrauterine device is inserted along with postoperative administration of high doses of estrogen followed by progestin. A relook hysteroscopy is done after 3 months to remove the IUD and assess for the need for further adhesiolysis.

Asherman's syndrome is a complex problem, which if tackled properly can lead to very gratifying and satisfying results in both restoration of menses and pregnancy for patients.

A bit-like Incontinence surgeries your best shot is with the first hysteroscopy if done properly.

Photo showing single anteroposterior adhesion in upper uterine cavity **(Fig. 8)** (Mild Asherman's syndrome).

Photo showing tubular cavity with adhesions obliterating more than 2/3rds of cavity **(Fig. 9)**.

Scissors

This is the safest technique for mechanically cutting adhesions and is central to our management approach. It effectively severs the adhesions while minimizing collateral damage, which could otherwise result from

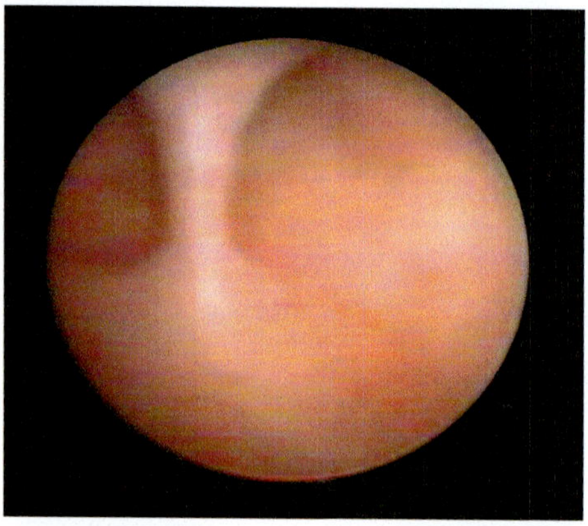

Fig. 8: Mild Asherman's syndrome (single anteroposterior adhesion in upper uterine cavity).

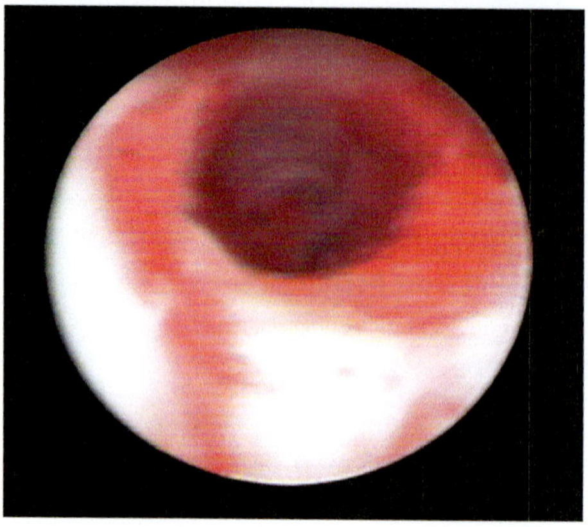

Fig. 9: Tubular cavity with adhesions obliterating more than 2/3rds of cavity.

the use of electrical or energy-based devices. Additionally, any perforation complications that arise during surgery with scissors are generally straightforward and easier to manage compared to more complex issues that may occur with other methods.

Laser

The Nd:YAG laser delivers energy via a fiber inserted through an operating hysteroscope, vaporizing tissue to a depth of 5–6 mm.

STEM CELL TREATMENT IN ASHERMAN'S SYNDROME

Endometrial regeneration using stem cell therapy has been explored in both animal models and small experimental human studies. Bone marrow-derived stem cells, mesenchymal stem cells, and autologous menstrual blood-derived stromal cells have been investigated. Various methods of application have been tried, including infusion into spiral arterioles via catheters, transmyometrial injection into the subendometrial area, and direct instillation of stromal cells into the uterine cavity after endometrial scratching.

In animal studies, stem cells arranged in spheroids were successful in repairing damaged endometrium. In a study by Singh et al. five out of six women resumed menstruation after treatment. Santa Maria et al. treated 15 women with AS, resulting in increased endometrial thickness and regular menstruation through hormone replacement therapy; four women conceived, with one successful live birth. In another study by Tan et al., seven women with refractory AS were treated with autologous menstrual blood-derived stromal cells, leading to improved endometrial thickness. Three patients conceived, with one ongoing pregnancy.

Further randomized trials are required to determine the potential clinical role of stem cell therapy in treating AS.

CONCLUSION

The prevention and treatment of Asherman's syndrome remain challenging, as the condition occurs sporadically after pregnancy termination or following the evacuation of a recently pregnant uterus. Emphasizing the importance of effective contraception is crucial in reducing the number of legal abortions. When abortion is medically indicated, medical termination is preferable, as it decreases the need for surgical evacuation and re-evacuation, which may lower the risk of developing intrauterine adhesions.

If evacuation of retained products of conception (RPOC) is required, it is essential to proceed gently to avoid the need for re-evacuation, which increases the likelihood of AS. In cases involving RPOC, hysteroscopy is preferred over curettage, as it carries a significantly lower risk of inducing intrauterine adhesions and is more effective at ensuring complete removal.

AS should be suspected if a patient experiences changes in menstrual patterns, menstrual pain, or infertility following intrauterine procedures. In some instances, saline-infusion ultrasonography may reveal defects in the uterine cavity. If AS is suspected, hysteroscopy should be performed to separate adhesions, preferably without the use of electric current, or using bipolar current to minimize complications.

To prevent the recurrence of adhesions, the use of balloon catheters or nonhormonal intrauterine devices (IUCDs) is recommended. Low-dose estrogen therapy may also be beneficial as a complementary treatment. AS is relatively rare and the surgery to treat it is complex, so severe cases should be referred to specialized centers where surgeons are experienced in advanced intrauterine surgery.

SUGGESTED READING

1. Asherman JG. Traumatic intra-uterine adhesions. J Obstet Gynaecol Br Emp. 1950;57(6):892-6. doi: 10.1111/j.1471-0528.1950.tb06053.x. [DOI] [PubMed] [Google Scholar]
2. Conforti A, Mollo A, Placido GD, Magos A. The management of Asherman syndrome: a review of literature. Reprod Biol Endocrinol 2013;11:118. doi: 10.1186/1477-7827-11-118.
3. Deans R, Vancaillie T, Ledger W, et al. Live birth rate and obstetrics complications following the hysteroscopic management of intrauterine adhesions including Asherman syndrome. Hum Reprod. 2018;33:1847-53.
4. Domnina A, Novikova P, Obidina J, et al. Human mesenchymal stem cells in spheroids improve fertility in model animals with damaged endometrium. Stem Cell Res Ther. 2018;9(1):50. doi: 10.1186/s13287-018-0801-9. [DOI] [PMC free article] [PubMed] [Google Scholar]
5. Dreisler E, Kjer JJ. Asherman's syndrome: current perspectives on diagnosis and management. Int J Womens Health. 2019;11:191-8. doi: 10.2147/IJWH.S165474
6. Hooker AB, de Leeuw R, van de Ven PM, et al. Prevalence of intrauterine adhesions after the application of hyaluronic acid gel after dilatation and curettage in women with at least one previous curettage: short-term outcomes of a multicenter, prospective randomized controlled trial. Fertil Steril. 2017;107(5):1223-31. doi: 10.1016/j.fertnstert.2017.02.113. [DOI] [PubMed] [Google Scholar].
7. Nagori CB, Panchal SY, Patel H. Endometrial regeneration using autologous adult stem cells followed by conception by in vitro fertilization in a patient of severe Asherman's syndrome. J Human Reprod Sci. 2011;4(1):43-8. doi: 10.4103/0974-1208.82360. [DOI] [PMC free article] [PubMed] [Google Scholar]
8. Singh N, Mohanty S, Seth T, Shankar M, Bhaskaran S, Dharmendra S. Autologous stem cell transplantation in refractory Asherman's syndrome: a novel cell based therapy. J Hum Reprod Sci. 2014;7(2):93-8. doi: 10.4103/0974-1208.138864. [DOI] [PMC free article] [PubMed] [Google Scholar]
9. Van Der Pas HV, Vancaillie T. Manual of Hysteroscopy. Amsterdam, the Netherlands: Elsevier, 2009.
10. Wamsteker K. European Society for Hysteroscopy (ESH) Classification;1989.

10 CHAPTER

Hysteroscopic Management of Isthmocele

Amogh Chimote

INTRODUCTION

An isthmocele is a discontinuity or anechoic gap in the anterior uterine wall in a previous cesarean scar.[1] *A* isthmocele *is also called as "uterine niche" or cesarean scar defect and these terms are mutually exchangeable.*

The presence of isthmocele was first described by Morris in 1955 in a study of 51 hysterectomy specimens in order to determine the pathological changes in the uterus with cesarean scar. of This entity was first described by this entity was first described by Morris in 1995 who studied a series of 51 hysterectomy specimens to define the pathological changes at the cesarean scar.[2] The development of isthmocele may be attributed to improper healing of the uterine incision at the isthmic level.[3]

Over the years, there have been various techniques for diagnosis like transvaginal sonography (TVS), magnetic resonance imaging (MRI), 3D-TVS saline infusion sonography (SIS), hysterosalpingography (HSG) and even hysteroscopy. Similarly depending on the size, position and symptomatology the modality of correction may change and can range from vaginal route, laparoscopic, hysteroscopic or even open laparotomy. In this chapter, we will be dealing with the role of hysteroscopy in management of uterine niche, its advantages, disadvantages, its place in restoring fertility, management of menstrual bleeding, instrumentation and the techniques for correction.

PREVALENCE

The prevalence of isthmocele may be varied and may range from as low as 6.9–69% with symptoms ranging from abnormal menstrual bleeding (AUB), postmenstrual or intermittent bleeding. It may lead to complications like scar ectopic pregnancies, severe-to-mild dysmenorrhea, isthmocele cysts or abscess formation.[4] Around 60% of women with cesarean delivery may develop a niche and around 25% of them may have a large defect with residual myometrial thickness (RMT) <3 mm.[5]

PATHOPHYSIOLOGY

The development of isthmocele is attributed to poor healing at the cesarean scar site which may be a result of certain risk factors **(Table 1)**. Four different hypotheses were proposed by Vervoort et al., which were: (1) Incision at lower level on cervix; (2) Incomplete surgical closure; (3) Ventral adhesion between the incision and anterior abdominal wall; (4) patient factors like wound healing and hemostasias.

DIAGNOSIS

Transvaginal ultrasound and saline infusion sonography (SIS) are primary imaging modalities used to identify isthmocele, often followed by hysteroscopy for direct visualization. A 3D ultrasound helps in further localization and exact position and volume of the isthmocele which may help in deciding the route of surgical correction **(Table 2)**.

TABLE 1: Risk factors for developing isthmocele.[7]

Risk factors for isthmocele	*Specifications*	*Comments*
Surgery-related factors	Cervical location of the uterine incision	Poor healing due to secretion of mucus from the endocervical glands
	Incomplete closure of uterine wall	May lead to formation of defects
	Single layer closure	Debatable cause, requires further studies, but few studies indicate that it may be one of the reasons
	Locking of sutures	Hypoxia of the tissues may lead to improper healing
	Postoperative infection	Tissue hypoxia due to poor vascularity and healing
Patient-related factors	Individual healing factors	Healing may differ from patient to patient
	Complications of pregnancy like gestational diabetes mellitus	Causative factor for inflammation, hence poor healing
	Number of cesarean	More than three sections: definitely causes niche formation
	Uterine position	More likely in retroverted uteri

TABLE 2: Diagnostic tools for isthmocele and its efficacy.[8]

Diagnostic modality	*Sensitivity*	*Specificity*	*Advantages*
Transvaginal ultrasound	80–90%	85–95%	Noninvasive, accessible
SIS	90–95%	90–97%	Enhanced visualization of niche
Hysteroscopy	100%	100%	Direct visualization and treatment

TABLE 3: Criteria required for diagnosis of cesarean scar disorder and conditions that should be ruled out before confirming the diagnosis.

Diagnostic criteria	*RoA, %*	*Conditions to exclude*	*RoA, %*
Minimum of three regular menstrual cycles after CD before diagnosis can be made	93.5	Cervical dysplasia	74.2
A patient needs to be premenopausal	100	Vaginal/uterine infections	74.2
The complaints of a symptomatic niche should start after a CD or should worsen significantly after a CD	80.6	Other uterine intracavitary pathology	93.5
A patient can be cured from a symptomatic niche (this does not mean that all symptomatic niche should be treated)	87.1	Other causes of postmenstrual spotting (such as continuous oral contraceptive use or intrauterine device)	80.6
NA	NA	Anovulatory cycles	100

(CD: cesarean delivery; NA: not applicable; RoA: rate of agreement)

A hysteroscopic examination typically reveals a niche or pouch in the anterior uterine wall, which may range from a few millimeters to several centimeters in size. Depending on the symptoms, RMT, and future prospects of fertility, the laparoscopic, vaginal or hysteroscopic route of correction may be chosen **(Table 3)**.

Although TVS is a noninvasive method of diagnosing the niche, hysteroscopy is the most reliable modality to diagnose as well as treatment of the pathology in the same setting.

IMPORTANT DEFINITIONS, CLASSIFICATION, MEASUREMENTS AND RELEVANCE

According to Jordan et al. who studied the niche according to Delphi procedure have given certain definitions for classification of the niche.[9]

A niche is always exclusively noted on the anterior isthmic region and can range from a few millimeters to as large as few centimeters. A niche can be classified as **(Figs. 1 to 3)**:

- Simple niche
- Simple niche with one branch
- Complex niche (with more than one branch)

A branch was agreed to be a thinner part of the main niche, which is directed towards the serosa and has a width smaller than that of the main niche and should always be recorded.[8]

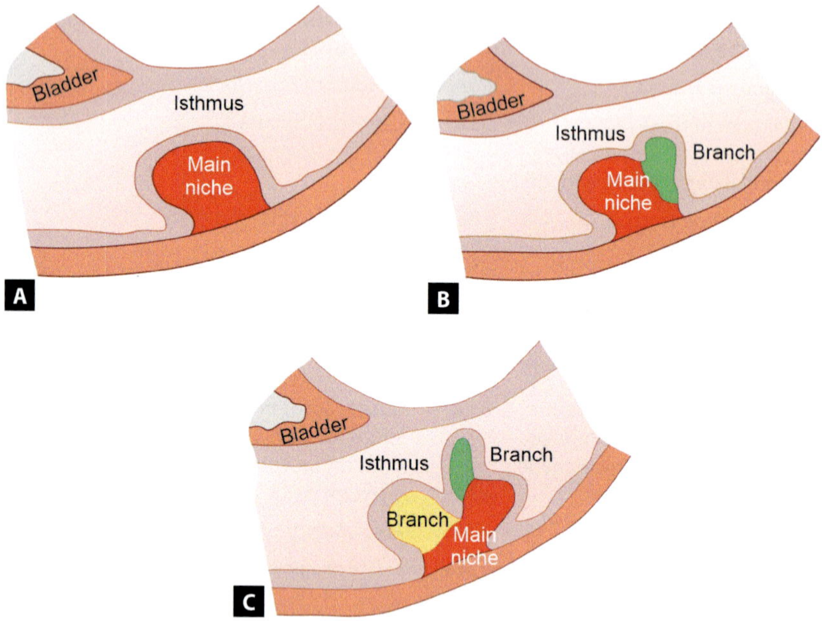

Figs. 1A to C: Types of isthmocele or niche can be broadly classified as: Simple niche (A); Simple niche with one branch; (B) Complex niche (C).[9]

SURGICAL MANAGEMENT

Once the diagnosis is established and the niche classified accordingly, the next step is the surgical intervention to repair the defect. Hysteroscopy, although a relatively easier option for management has its own shortcoming when it comes to correction of the defect.

Contraindications for Hysteroscopic Repair of Niche

- Large niche (>50% defect)
- Residual myometrial thickness <2.5 mm and <3.5 mm (future fertility)
- Complex niche

Hysteroscopic Technique

Hysteroscopic management involves resecting the fibrotic tissue, granulomatous tissue as well as the fibrotic rings within the isthmocele and restoring normal endometrial contour. The technique includes the following steps:

Preoperative Assessment

A detailed evaluation with imaging is essential to determine the extent of the defect. Measurements of the isthmocele depth, width, and residual

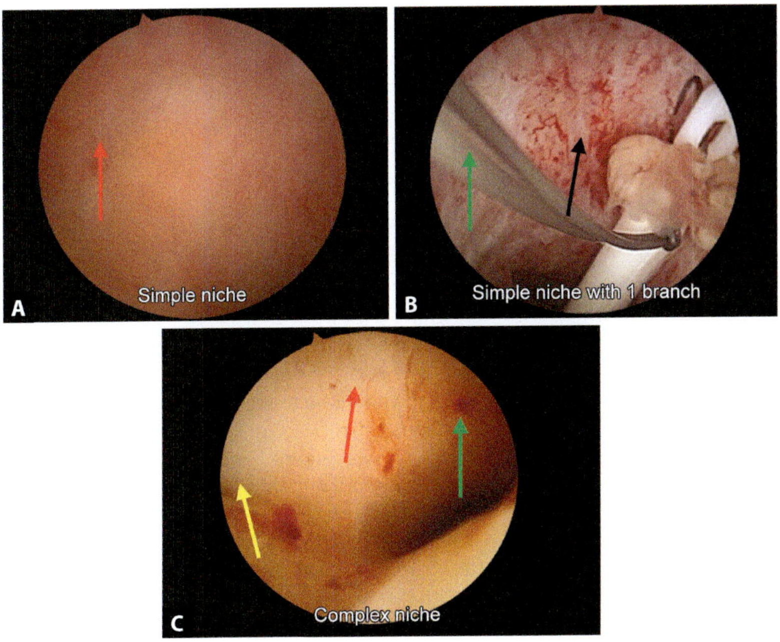

Figs. 2A to C: Images of classification of niche showing various depths and branches: (A) A simple niche with a single defective areas at the isthmus with depth <1 cm; (B) A simple cyst with 1 additional branch which also shows granulomatous growth around the Mirena®, which was the cause of recurrent menstrual bleeding; (C) A large defect with more than 1 branch and a depth >1 cm. (Red arrow: main Defect; Green arrow: branch of isthmocele; Yellow arrow: 2nd branch of isthmocele)
Images Courtesy: Dr Amogh Chimote, Vaunshdhara Fertility Centre, Nagpur, Maharashtra, India.

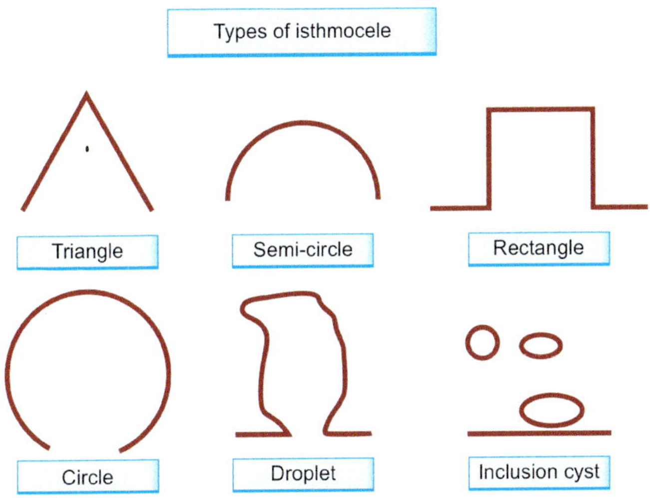

Fig. 3: Different shapes of isthmoceles that can be seen on imaging.

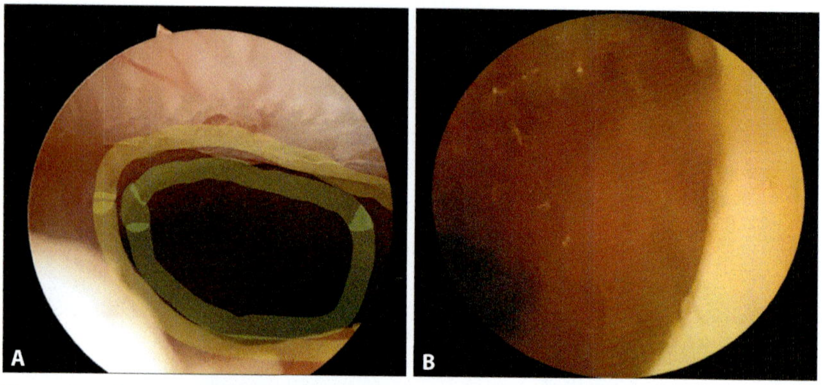

Figs. 4A and B: Histological os (yellow) and anatomical os (green), also labeled as outer ring (cervix, yellow) and inner ring (isthmus, green).
Images Courtesy: Figure (A) Dr Amogh Chimote; Figure (B) Dr Sandesh Kade (https://youtu.be/9CdIMkICoq0).

myometrial thickness (RMT) are crucial in planning the surgery by a 2D–3D TVS **(Figs. 4A and B)**.

Procedure:

- Under general anesthesia, a hysteroscope is inserted vaginoscopically and the endocervical canal is negotiated by following the grooves of the endocervical glands.
- Internal os is identified and without negotiating the os, we try to identify the histological and the anatomical os.
- It is important to identify and distinguish the 2 rings (green and yellow in the above **Figure 4A**) as the pouch or defect between these 2 rings is the isthmocele.
- The principle of the technique is to create a smooth transition so as to create regular contours which will avoid accumulation of blood leading to infection, hence the symptoms.
- There are 2 slopes emanating from the inner ring that is the upper slope (area in red in **Figure 5A**) and the lower slope (area in yellow in the **Figure 5B**)
- Resectoscope with Collin's knife is introduced and releasing incisions given till we reach the floor of the isthmocele. Simultaneous incisions are given over the inner and outer ring so as to maintain a proper plane **(Figs. 6A and B)**.
- Releasing incision on the roof or inner ring corresponding with incision of the base **(Fig. 7)**.
- The releasing incision work as a guideline and limit of the resection of tissue so that the entire defect becomes like a smooth cone **(Fig. 8)**.

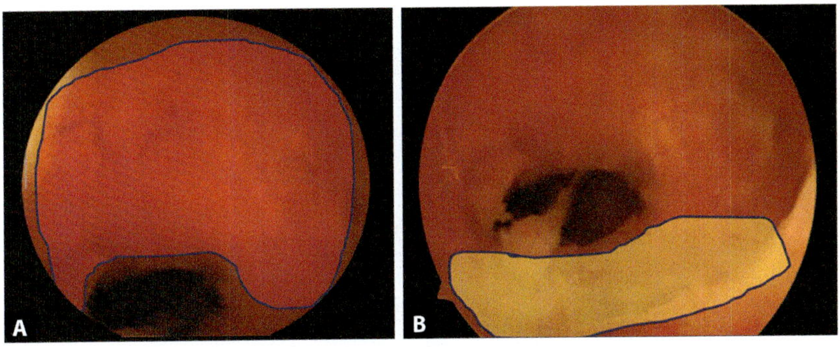

Figs. 5A and B: Complete anatomy of a simple niche with the red area showing the ventral slope while the yellow area shows the dorsal slope. These are the areas which are generally resected hysteroscopically to correct the defect.

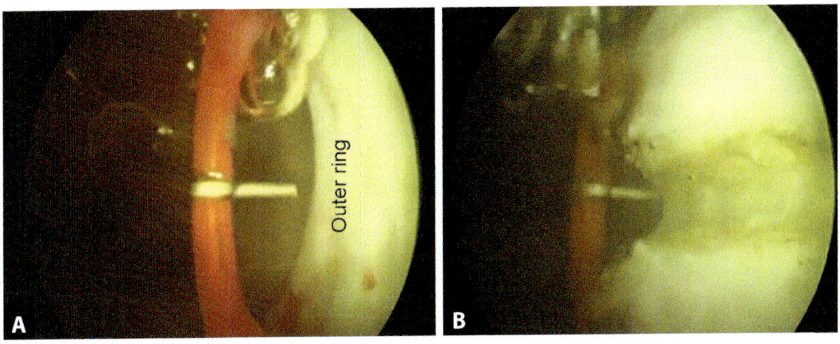

Figs. 6A and B: (A) Use of Collin's knife to incise outer ring simultaneously till the base or floor of the isthmocele; (B) Incision in progress with a resectoscope.

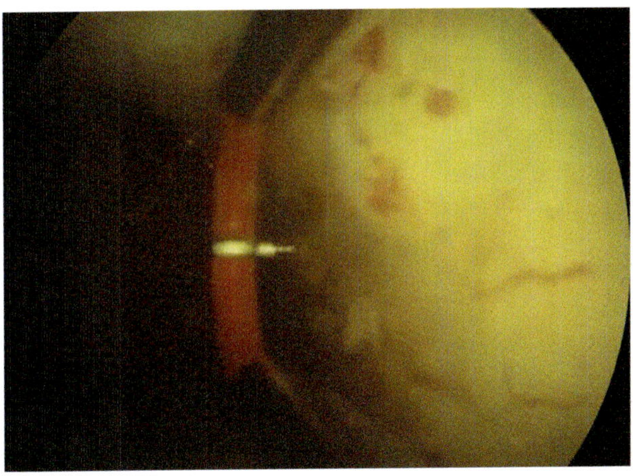

Fig. 7: Releasing incision on the roof or inner ring corresponding with incision of the base.

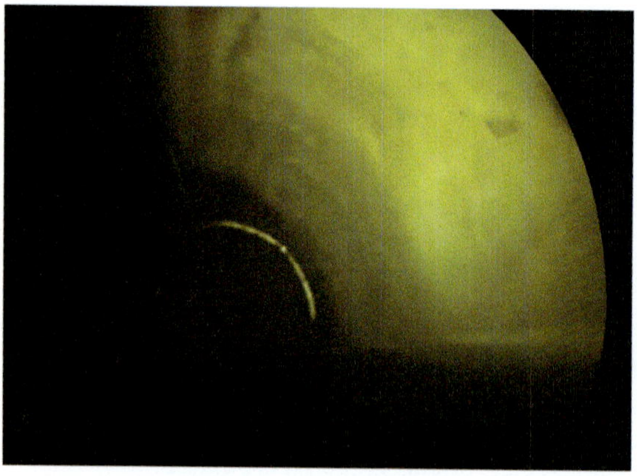

Fig. 8: Loop electrode is used to flatten the ring till the required depth or just reaching till the depth of the defect.

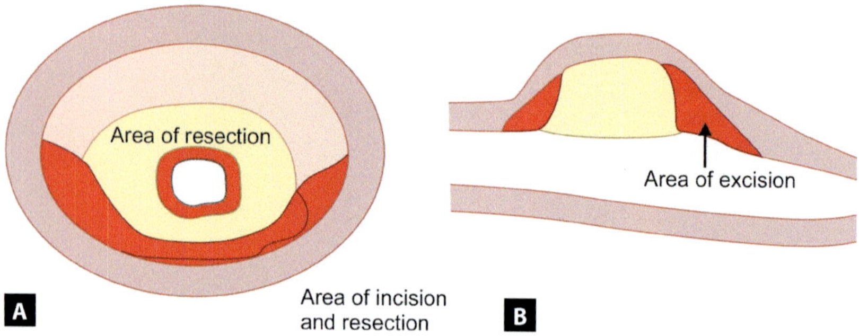

Figs. 9A and B: Schematic representation of hysteroscopic view. (A) The area in the red is the areas of excision with a Collin's knife, while the area in light yellow represents the areas of resection with a loop; (B) Schematic diagram (Sagittal section) showing resection of the area in red with a loop in order to flatten the defect.

- Loop electrode is used to flatten the ring till the required depth or just reach till the depth of the defect so as to get a uniform surface from inner to the outer ring **(Figs. 9A and B)**.

An important point to remember is always visualize the internal os clearly to stay in the right plane and direction and take thin slices when using a Collin's knife. It is always better to under correct to avoid future chances of perforation as well as injury to the bladder. What the surgeon must bear in mind is that the myometrial thickness is in millimeters and hence there are higher chances of injury to the bladder or bowel due to thermal injury from the resectoscope.

There has been a description of newer techniques which may differ from the above one only slightly, but the principle remains the same, i.e., creating a uniform passage or pathway to avoid accumulation of blood.

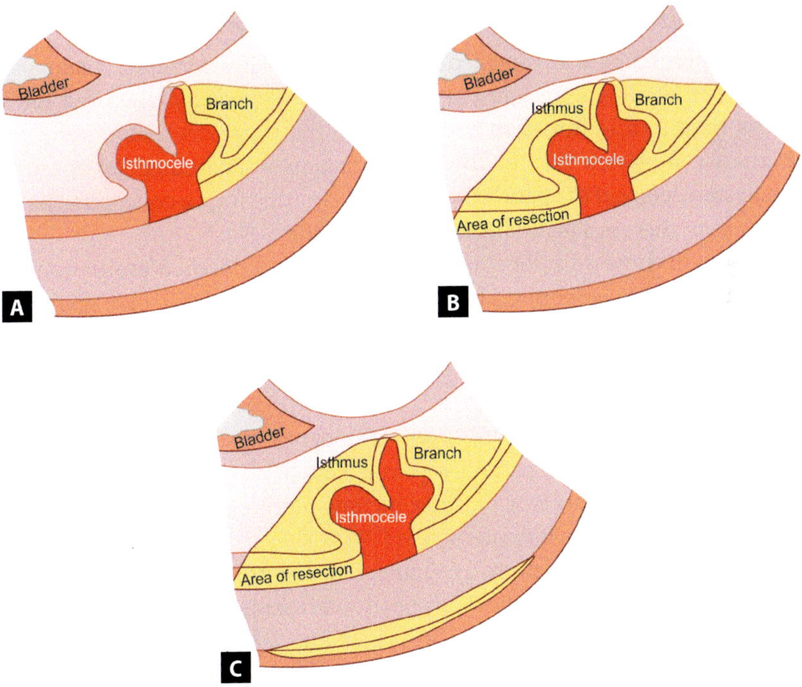

Figs. 10A to C: (A) Fabre's technique in which only the lower part or outer ring is resected; (B) Gubbini's technique in which the inner as well as the posterior ring is resected; (C) 360º technique in which along with inner and outer ring the posterior aspect is also resected. The red area shows the isthmocele, the yellow shows the areas of resection.

TABLE 4: Comparative success rates of different surgical modalities.[12]

Surgical method	*Symptomatic relief (%)*	*Pregnancy rates (%)*	*Complication rates (%)*
Hysteroscopic resection	85	52	2
Laparoscopic repair	90	65	8
Combined hystero-laparoscopic	92	68	6

These techniques are Fabre's technique,[3] Gubbini's Technique,[10] and channel like 360º technique[11] **(Figs. 10A to C)**.

OUTCOMES AND SUCCESS RATES

Recent studies indicate that hysteroscopic resection of isthmocele provides symptomatic relief in over 85% of patients. A *2022 meta-analysis* found that women treated with hysteroscopic repair had a *76% improvement in postmenstrual spotting* and a *52% success rate in achieving pregnancy* within 12 months of the procedure **(Table 4)**.

CHALLENGES IN SURGICAL MANAGEMENT

While hysteroscopy is advantageous for its minimal invasiveness, challenges arise when dealing with large or deep defects, especially when the RMT is less than 2 mm, hence in such cases some surgeons recommend an alternative approach like laparoscopic or vaginal or combined laparoscopy and hysteroscopy, if the patient is especially desiring future conception as in these cases, there is a higher risk of uterine rupture.

Owing to these complications, a complete and detailed evaluation by imaging modality is required before planning hysteroscopic management. Careful consideration and counseling are a must.

LONG-TERM FOLLOW-UP AND COMPLICATIONS

Postoperative follow-up includes repeat imaging to assess the restoration of uterine anatomy and patient-reported outcomes. Complications from hysteroscopic repair are rare but may include uterine perforation, excessive bleeding, and adhesion formation.

A 2021 retrospective study by Vitale et al. reported that *98% of patients experienced no major complications* posthysteroscopic repair. However, the risk of recurrence of isthmocele persists in about *10% of cases*, particularly in women who undergo repeat cesarean sections.[13]

NEWER APPROACHES

Advancements in laser-assisted hysteroscopic techniques have shown promising results. This involves a combined approach of hysteroscopy and laparoscopy with the use of near infrared vision (available in latest high-definition camera system) CO_2 laser operated by a robotic arm. The hysteroscopy is done and transillumination is performed which is then visualized under the infrared filter to identify the extent of the defect. The defect is then excised with laser and good margins are created. After the complete excision the hysteroscope is removed and the defect is sutured with barbed sutures or in 2 layers. After the procedure, a catheter (Oley's/Malecot's cathter) is placed to avoid adhesion formation and stenosis.[14]

Currently, there is no gold standard technique for management of niche but this combined technique seems to be the most efficacious way of correcting the defect as it ensures complete clearance of the fibrous tissue and good strength to the scar in cases where future fertility is a prospect.[14]

CONCLUSION

Hysteroscopic management of isthmocele offers a safe, minimally invasive option for symptomatic women, providing relief from postmenstrual bleeding and may help improving fertility outcomes in selective cases. Continued advancements in hysteroscopic techniques, such as the integration of laser technology and 3D visualization, are poised to improve surgical success rates and reduce complications. Long-term studies are required to further refine these techniques and ensure optimal outcomes for patients.

REFERENCES

1. Gubbini G, Casadio P, Marra E. Resectoscopic correction of the "isthmocele" in women with postmenstrual abnormal uterine bleeding and secondary infertility. J Minim Invasive Gynecol. 2008;15(2):172-5. doi: 10.1016/j.jmig.2007.10.004. PMID: 18312986.
2. Morris H. Surgical pathology of the lower uterine segment caesarean section scar: is the scar a source of clinical symptoms? Int J Gynecol Pathol. 1995;14(1): 16-20. doi: 10.1097/00004347-199501000-00004. PMID:7883420.
3. Dominguez JA, Pacheco LA, Moratalla E, Carugno JA, Carrera M, Perez-Milan F, Caballero M, Alcázar JL. Diagnosis and management of isthmocele (Cesarean scar defect): a SWOT analysis. Ultrasound Obstet Gynecol. 2023;62: 336-44. https://doi.org/10.1002/uog.26171.
4. Tower AM, Frishman GN. Cesarean scar defects: an underrecognized cause of abnormal uterine bleeding and other gynecologic complications. J Minim Invasive Gynecol. 2013;20(5):562-72. doi: 10.1016/j.jmig.2013.03.008. Epub 2013 May 14. PMID: 23680518.
5. Stagwee SI, Jordans IPM, van der Voet LF, et al. Single-versus double-layer closure of the caesarean (uterine) scar in the prevention of gynaecological symptoms in relation to niche development—the 2Close study: a multicentre randomised controlled trial. BMC Pregnancy Childbirth. 2019;19(1):85. doi: 10.1186/s12884-019-2221-y. PMID: 30832681; PMCID: PMC6399840.
6. Vervoort A, Vissers J, Hehenkamp W, Brölmann H, Huirne J. The effect of laparoscopic resection of large niches in the uterine caesarean scar on symptoms, ultrasound findings and quality of life: a prospective cohort study. BJOG. 2018;125(3):317-25. doi: 10.1111/1471-0528.14822. Epub 2017 Aug 28. PMID: 28703935; PMCID: PMC5811817.
7. Drizi A. Isthmocele: New Insights and Review. The Trocar, 2023;(1) Article 013. https://doi.org/10.36205/trocar1.2023013.
8. Meuleman SJMK, Murji A, van den Bosch T, Donnez O, Grimbizis G, Saridogan E, Chantraine F, Bourne T, Timmerman D, Huirne JAF, de Leeuw RA; CSDi Study Group. Definition and Criteria for Diagnosing Cesarean Scar Disorder. JAMA Netw Open. 2023;6(3):e235321. doi: 10.1001/jamanetworkopen.2023.5321. PMID: 36988956; PMCID: PMC10061236.
9. Jordans, IPM, de Leeuw, RA, Stegwee SI, et al. Sonographic examination of uterine niche in non-pregnant women: A modified Delphi procedure. Ultrasound in Obstetrics & Gynecology. 2018;52(1):131-9. https://doi.org/10.1002/uog.19049.
10. Gubbini G, Casadio P, Marra E. Resectoscopic correction of the "isthmocele" in women with postmenstrual abnormal uterine bleeding and secondary infertility. J Minim Invasive Gynecol. 2008;15(2):172-5. doi: 10.1016/j.jmig.2007.10.004. PMID: 18312986.

11. Casadio P, Gubbini G, Morra C, Franchini M, Paradisi R, Seracchioli R. Channel-like 360° isthmocele treatment with a 16F mini-resectoscope: a step-by-step technique. J Minim Invasive Gynecol. 2019;26(7):1229-30. doi: 10.1016/j.jmig.2019.04.024. Epub 2019 May 3. PMID: 31059782.
12. Verberkt Carry, et al. Fertility and pregnancy outcomes after a uterine niche resection in women with and without infertility: a systematic review and meta-analysis. F&S Reviews. 2022;3(3):174-89.
13. Vitale SG, Ludwin A, Vilos GA, Török P, Tesarik J, Vitagliano A, Lasmar RB, Chiofalo B. From hysteroscopy to laparoendoscopic surgery: what is the best surgical approach for symptomatic isthmocele? A systematic review and meta-analysis. Archives of Gynecology and Obstetrics. 2020;301(1):33-52. https://doi.org/10.1007/s00404-020-05438-0.
14. Walker Z, Gargiulo A. Near-infrared and hysteroscopy-guided robotic excision of uterine isthmocele with laser fiber: a novel high-precision technique. Fertility and Sterility. 2023;120(5):1081-3. https://doi.org/10.1016/j.fertnstert.2023.08.006.

11

CHAPTER

Hysteroscopic Management of Subtle Lesions in Infertile Patients

Salvatore Giovanni Vitale, Stefania Saponara, Gaetano Riemma, Manoj Chellani

INTRODUCTION

While many intrauterine pathologies are easily recognized and treated during in-office hysteroscopy, in some cases, even the most experienced operator can miss the diagnosis of an intracavitary lesion which can lead to infertility issues.[1]

Relative to infertility, a subtle lesion is an abnormal condition of uterine cavity that should be treated to increase fertility chances. However, a clear definition of "subtle" lesion is far from being stated, since not everybody calls the same lesion in the same way.[2]

Moreover, there are cases in which, even if recognized, a subtle lesion of the uterus is classified as "normal" and remains untreated.[3] For this reason, a lack of uniform, standardized and universally accepted terminology is the greatest detrimental for the diagnosis and treatment of such pathologies.[4]

Considering the above, there are several subtle causes of infertility that could be resolved using hysteroscopy.[5] They are mainly categorized in anatomical (i.e., dysmorphic uteri), myometrial (i.e., intramural and submucosal uterine myomas) and endometrial (i.e., chronic endometritis) dysfunctions. In addition, iatrogenic lesions to the uterine cavity can also cause undiagnosed or misdiagnosed reproductive issues.[5,6,9-13]

Adjuvated by ultrasonography, a modern "one-stop" hysteroscopic approach, in which the operator can diagnose and treat also the most subtle lesion, is a feasible way to resolve infertility problems that are related to a subtle, not self-evident, cause.[1,7]

CERVICAL ABNORMALITIES

The vast majority of cervical lesions are not linked to infertility issues; however, some lesions are commonly accounted for recurrent pregnancy losses. In particular, first trimester losses are mainly associated with implantation issues, which could be related to an altered endometrial microenvironment. In such scenario, cervical polyps and cervicitis are mostly recognized as leading factors. Meanwhile, for late pregnancy losses, cervical incompetence is considered the leading cause. The following organic lesions are subtle causes or cervix-related subfertility issues, especially for late pregnancy losses.[8]

Cervical Leiomyomas

Cervical leiomyomas **(Figs. 1A and B)** account for less than 5% of uterine myomas and are divided into two types according to the location, (1) submucosal (with an intracervical location), or (2) subserosal (with an extracervical location). They are clonal benign proliferation of smooth muscle cells, usually, they can be associated with abnormal vaginal bleeding, dyspareunia and infertility. Cervical myomas have to be differentiated, especially in the pedunculated shape, from large polyps or neoplasms protruding from the uterine cavity.[14,15] Often, transvaginal ultrasound is necessary to better define the size and location of the lesion, evaluating the relation that it can have with closer organs such as the bladder, ureter, and rectum. Office hysteroscopic treatment can be performed in case of small, pedunculated leiomyomas, while in case of myomatous lesions of large size and/or those presenting an intramural part, they should be treated by resectoscopic surgery in an operating room setting.[16] The presence of cervical leiomyomas is related with poor reproductive and obstetric outcomes, with increased early and late pregnancy loss rates, making of them a subtle cause of subfertility.

Cervical and Vaginal Endometriosis

Cervical or vaginal endometriosis is an uncommon benign condition that may appear at endoscopic evaluation as a bluish red or bluish-black lesion **(Fig. 2)**. This condition can be extremely heterogeneous: it can be

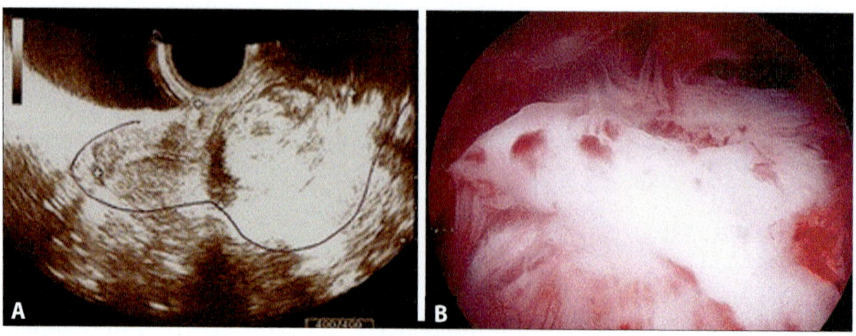

Figs. 1A and B: Ultrasonographic (A) and hysteroscopic (B) image of an endocervical myoma.

Source: Bigatti G, Ferrario C, Rosales M, Baglioni A, Bianchi S. A 4-cm G2 cervical submucosal myoma removed with the IBS® integrated Bigatti shaver. Gynecol Surg. 2012;9(4):453-6. doi: 10.1007/s10397-012-0737-5).

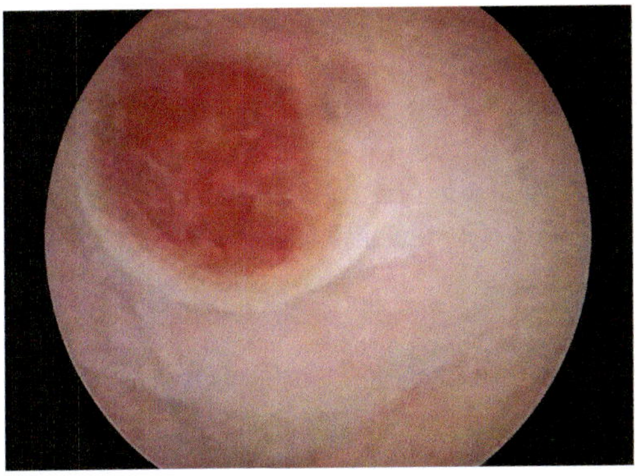

Fig. 2: Vaginal endometriosis.

Source: Nappi C, Di Spiezio Sardo A. Rare and difficult-to-interpret hysteroscopic findings. In: Nappi C, Di Spiezio Sardo A (Eds). State-of-the-Art Hysteroscopic Approaches to Pathologies of the Genital tract. Tuttlingen: Endo-Press; 2014.

asymptomatic or cause symptoms such as persistent postcoital bleeding, intermenstrual bleeding, or symptomatology not dissimilar to that of pelvic endometriosis. Cervical endometriosis has been accounted to be a possible factor of subtle infertility, although the noncommon occurrence of such localization unveils the need for further research to improve the state of knowledge.[17]

MORPHOLOGICAL ABNORMALITIES

Uterine and cervical morphological anomalies also play a significant role in subtle infertility issues. As also mentioned in the previous chapters, a morphologically abnormal uterus or cervix can alter fertility in terms of recurrent pregnancy loss and primary or secondary infertility.[18]

While the presence of a uterine septum is easier to diagnose and treat, a uterus with a reduced global volume could be an undiagnosed, T-shaped, dysmorphic uterus.

On regards to dysmorphic uteri, according to the ESHRE/ESGE classification of Müllerian anomalies, a Class U1 anomaly has a regular uterine outline but an irregular uterine cavity, excluding the septa. This class includes three subtypes: "T-Shaped Uteri" (U1a) characterized by a narrow uterine cavity due to thickened lateral walls with a correlation 2/3 uterine corpus and 1/3 cervix; "infantilis uteri" (U1b), with a narrow cavity without thickened walls with a correlation of 1/3 uterine corpus and 2/3 cervix; and "others" (U1c) which contains all the minor uterine cavity deformities.[21]

Dysmorphic uteri prevalence has been underestimated because of many undiagnosed cases, leading to considering such anomalies a subtle infertility factor. Impaired uterine motility due to irregular and unnecessary myometrial contraction have been advocated as one the major issue for impaired fertility.[22] Improved examination methods and diagnostic standardization for dysmorphic uteri[23] enhanced the identification of these and other unknown anomalies.[24] Relative to these developments, reproductive outcomes after surgical correction of a dysmorphic uterus steadily improved, leading to increased uterine volume and normal morphology.[19] However, only few and sometimes small cohort studies show the impact of a regularized uterine cavity and volumes on reproductive and obstetric outcomes.[20]

However, it can be feasibly repaired by means of hysteroscopy and, in most patients, even in the office setting without anesthesia **(Figs. 3A to F)**.[25]

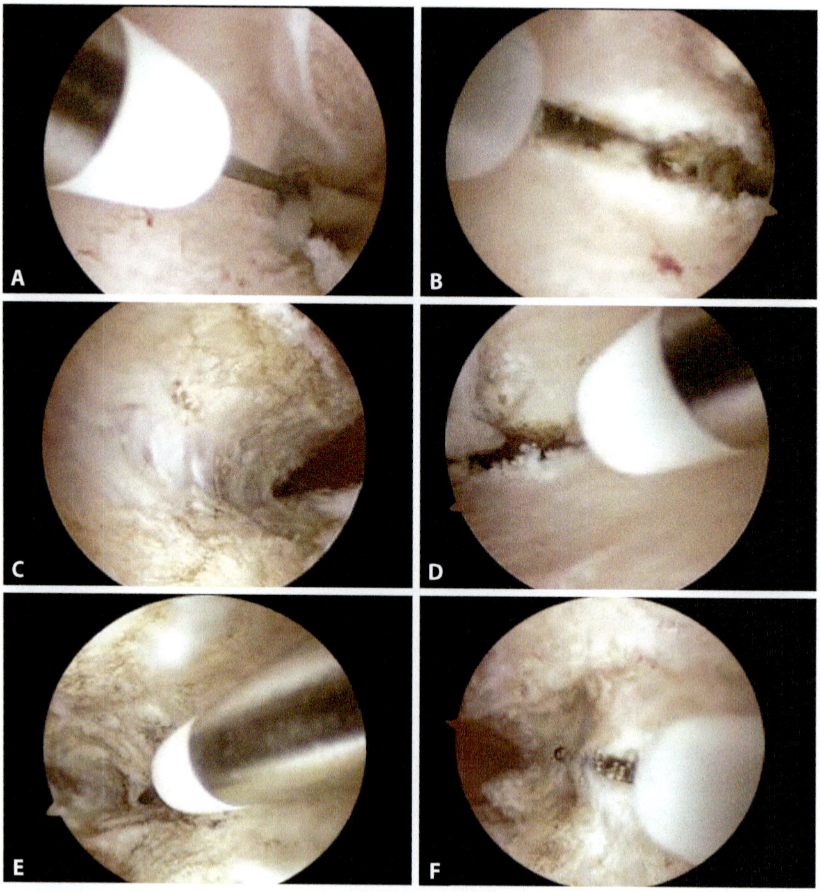

Figs. 3A to F: HOME-DU technique on a T-shaped (U1a) uterus. Superficial cuts on the uterine walls (A to F).

Source: Nappi C, Di Spiezio Sardo A. Rare and difficult-to-interpret hysteroscopic findings. In: Nappi C, Di Spiezio Sardo A (Eds). State-of-the-art hysteroscopic approaches to pathologies of the genital tract. Tuttlingen: Endo-Press; 2014. pp. 236-49.

It should be stressed that due to ethical constrains no randomized clinical trials or case-control studies that compare treatment to no treatment regimens are available.[26] However, the overall reproductive outcomes reported in several systematic reviews and meta-analyses, together with feasibility and cost-effectiveness analysis of hysteroscopic metroplasty, indicate its efficacy.[27]

The hysteroscopic management of Müllerian anomalies is also extensively described in the appropriate chapter.

ENDOMETRIAL ABNORMALITIES

Endometrial abnormalities account for the majority of uncommon or less common causes of subfertility among reproductive aged women. In this section, the most important subtle causes of infertility are summarized.

Chronic Endometritis

Chronic endometritis (CE) is a chronic condition characterized by subtle inflammation of the endometrium related to the infiltration of plasma cells in the endometrial stromal area **(Figs. 4A to D)**.[28-35] Although the clinical significance of CE has been object of several studies during the years, recent data have shown the potential adverse effects of CE on fertility; in particular, it seems to be associated with poor reproductive outcomes, including implantation failure and recurrent pregnancy loss, due to the inadequate microenvironment that interferes with normal implantation and endometrial receptivity.[36] CE has been included among subtle lesions due to several reasons. First, although standardized criteria are fundamental for diagnosis, some operators may judge the hysteroscopic view as non-pathological or vice versa. Similarly, sometimes CE is represented by unclear and shaded hysteroscopic images, which are frequently misdiagnosed or undiagnosed. For this reason, the gold standard for the diagnosis of CE is the histological detection of plasma cells in the stromal area of the endometrium in endometrial specimens and hysteroscopy can be considered a good tool for diagnosis of CE, considering its role not only in endometrial biopsy for the histological diagnosis but also in the macroscopical evaluation of usual CE findings such as presence of local or diffuse hyperemia, edema of the stroma and presence of micropolyps (less than 1 mm in size).[8] The treatment currently thought to be most effective for the recovery of fertility in CE is administration of oral antibiotics.[37]

Prolonged Hypoestrogenic Environment (Thin Endometrium)

A "Thin" endometrium is defined as an endometrium characterized by inadequate growth with subsequent adverse effect on reproductive

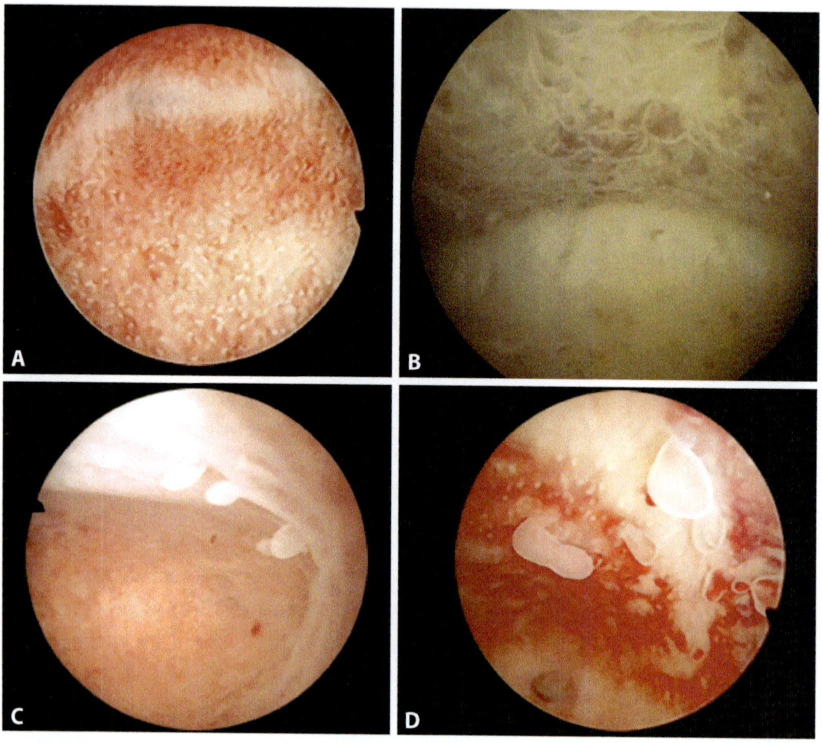

Figs. 4A to D: *Chronic endometritis:* Different hysteroscopic features of chronic endometritis. (A) Endometrial mucosa shows diffuse hyperemia, the hyperemic endometrium was flushed with a white central point, like "strawberry spots"; (B) Endometrial mucosa appears thickened, edematous, and focally hyperemic; (C) Endometrial surface is covered by sporadic micropolyps; (D) Endometrial mucosa shows diffuse hyperemia with multiple micropolyps.

Source: Song D, Li TC, Zhang Y, Feng X, Xia E, Huang X, Xiao Y. Correlation between hysteroscopy findings and chronic endometritis. Fertil Steril. 2019;111(4):772-9. doi: 10.1016/j.fertnstert.2018.12.007. Epub 2019 Jan 22.

performance **(Fig. 5)**,[37] considering that an adequate thickness of the endometrium is one of the main factors in implantation and pregnancy.[38] According to the most recent evidence, endometrial thickness under 7 mm would define a thin endometrium with compromised success rates.[39] The most frequent cause of thin endometrium lies in its surgical origin through the development of intrauterine adhesions (IUA), or to prolonged hypoestrogenic environment or also to radiotherapy below the diaphragm owing to malignancies. A possible validity of hysteroscopy in thin endometrium cases could be to diagnose a previously unrecognized uterine pathology, especially intrauterine adhesions produced by previous inflammatory processes, either with or without previous surgical trauma.[37] In case of IUA, hysteroscopic adhesiolysis should be performed to restore a

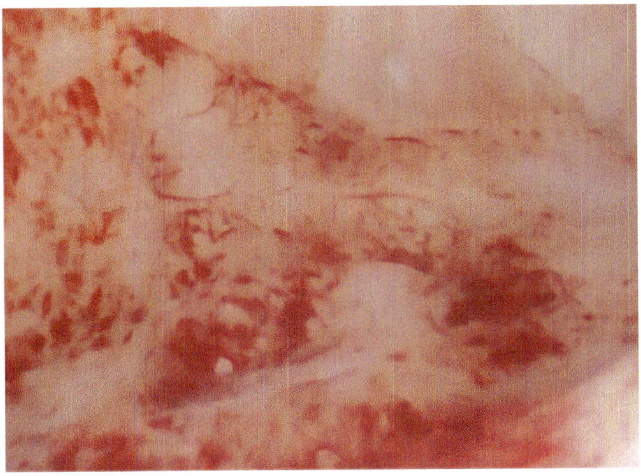

Fig. 5: Irregular "thin" endometrium with subendometrial hemorrhage.
Source: Adapted by permission from Springer Nature from Tinelli et al. Atlas of Hysteroscopy, 2020, Springer.

normal shape and volume of the uterine cavity; the hysteroscopic treatment can be performed in an outpatient setting, using miniaturized instruments, or may also involve the use of a classic resectoscope in the operating theater. An important step in this procedure is to prevent the recurrence of synechia: the hysteroscopic "second look" procedure performed within 1 month after surgery permit to evaluate the normalization of the uterine cavity, along with the option of an immediate lysis of any small remnants of synechiae. Moreover, based on the idea that separation of the endometrial layers after hysteroscopic surgery should help prevent the formation or recurrence of adhesions and promote physiologic endometrial regeneration, several barrier methods such as the placement of an IUD or a Foley catheter or intrauterine balloon (IUB) or the use of hyaluronic acid gel applied in the uterine cavity after completion of hysteroscopic synechiolysis have been evaluated in the literature.[33]

Endometrial Osseous Metaplasia

Endometrial osseous metaplasia **(Fig. 6)** is an uncommon entity, with nearly 200 cases reported in available literature. It is defined as the presence of mature or immature bone tissue in the endometrium.[50] Several authors incorrectly reported osseous metaplasia of the endometrium as endometrial ossification, ectopic intrauterine bone, or heterotopic intrauterine bone formation. Histopathologically, it varies from reactive to degenerative lesions. Moreover, it has been reported as a cause of secondary infertility after a spontaneous or provoked miscarriage.[50] Women with an endometrial

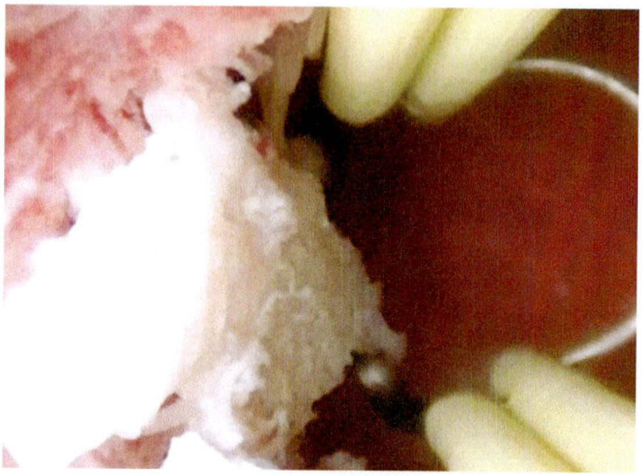

Fig. 6: Endometrial osseous metaplasia.
Source: Amodeo S, Iannone V, Borriello M, Giambanco L. Hysteroscopic management of endometrial osseous metaplasia mimicking a foreign body. J Minim Invasive Gynecol. 2021;28(10):1673-4.

osseous metaplasia shows normal and regular cyclical changes of the endometrium, as noticed in our case. It characteristically appears in women in their reproductive years, although, it has been reported in the menopausal years as well. A history of previous pregnancy is reported in >80% of the cases.[51] Hormonal or exogenous stimuli (intrauterine contraceptive device) are the main inducing, factors of endometrial metaplasias; rarely, some transformations have a mutational origin.[6] The removal of such lesion can be done in both the in-office and in-patient setting using mechanical forceps or bipolar electrodes. In case of larger osseous fragments, an in-patient resectoscopic approach should be preferred by the operator.[7]

OTHER SUBTLE LESIONS RELATED TO INFERTILITY

Although they do not represent a major and common issue for women's fertility, there are several iatrogenic, multifactorial, and tubal diseases that can lead to subtle reduction of fertility potential. Among those pathologies, it is mandatory to consider adenomyosis and several tubal factors.

Adenomyosis

Adenomyosis is defined as the presence of ectopic, non-neoplastic, endometrial glands and stroma in the myometrium, disorder that can anatomically manifest as one or a combination of thickening of the internal myometrium, areas of focal or diffuse disease, and involvement of the outer myometrium. Although evidence has been conflicting, there seems to be an overall negative impact of adenomyosis on fertility and on assisted reproductive technology outcomes **(Fig. 7)**.[40] The contribution of adenomyosis to infertility is

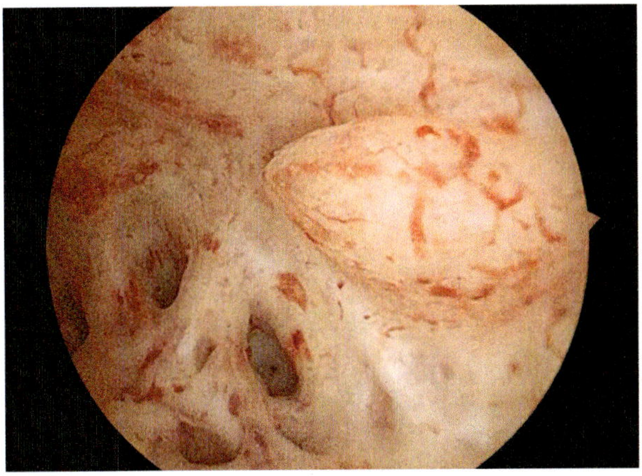

Fig. 7: Adenomyosis of the uterine cavity with ectopic glandular foci.
Source: Adapted by permission from Springer Nature from Tinelli et al. Atlas of Hysteroscopy, 2020, Springer.

believed to be linked to the change of the normal myometrial architecture and to the alteration of its function by dysfunctional uterine peristalsis and reduced endometrial receptivity. Hysteroscopy is considered an important adjunctive diagnostic procedure in the evaluation of adenomyosis as it offers the advantage of direct visualization of the uterine cavity and of some findings such as irregular endometrium with tiny openings on the endometrial surface, pronounced hypervascularization and hemorrhagic cystic lesions assuming a dark blue or chocolate-brown appearance that seems to be related to superficial adenomyosis.[33-38] Hysteroscopy allows also to obtain biopsy samples from the endometrium and underlying myometrium using mechanical instruments (biopsy or grasping forceps, scissors) or bipolar electrodes, or using an instrument called 'Spirotome' (Bioncise NV, Wellen, Belgium), that collecting samples from the subendometrial myometrium, giving an additional information regarding the penetration depth of the pathology.

As with diagnosis, hysteroscopy is not a first line treatment option for adenomyosis and should be used as a valid surgical therapy only in selected cases of superficial adenomyosis, as for evacuating cystic hemorrhagic lesions or enucleating superficial focal adenomyomas of less than 1.5 cm in diameter.[40-49]

Subtle Lesions of the Fallopian Tubes

Fallopian tube pathologies, including tubal blockage, acute and chronic salpingitis, hydrosalpinx, as well as peritubal adhesions, and salpingitis isthmica nodosa account for at least 30–40% of all infertility cases.[51-56]

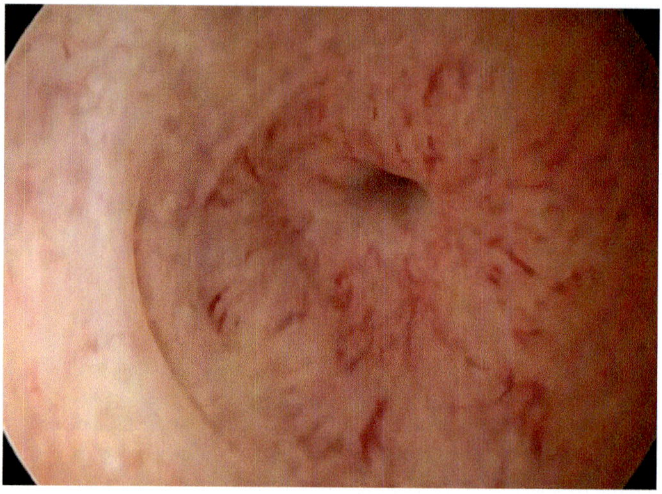

Fig. 8: The "tubal ostium Sunshine" for chronic salpingitis.
Source: Nappi C, Di Spiezio Sardo A. Rare and difficult-to-interpret hysteroscopic findings. In: Nappi C, Di Spiezio Sardo A (Eds). State-of-the-art hysteroscopic approaches to pathologies of the genital tract. Tuttlingen: Endo-Press; 2014. pp. 236-49.

Most commonly, fallopian tube occlusion is related to as pelvic inflammatory disease, typically caused by a sexually transmitted agent such as *Chlamydia trachomatis* or *Neisseria gonorrhoeae.*[52] In case of a regular morphology of the uterine cavity and regular endometrium, proximal tubal pathologies may be accounted as a leading cause. They can be considered subtle lesions since they are often misdiagnosed by the operator. Hysteroscopy is a trustful way to assess fallopian tubal patency and proximal pathologies. Hysteroscopic tubal assessment can be observational, such as the swirl test, or interventional, such as through air bubble infusion or methylene blue chromopertubation. Although laparoscopic chromopertubation will remain the gold standard hysteroscopic tubal patency assessment has the potential to be faster and more convenient and cost-effective, particularly in cases in which the women were already undergoing office hysteroscopy for uterine evaluation as part of their procreative evaluation.[57] In case of chronic salpingitis, its diagnostic confirmation involves multiple examinations, including sonography, cervicovaginal swab and lab test, hysteroscopy can be usefully included in its diagnostic work-up. The image resembles a hyperemic area patterned by radial arrangement of the vessels around the uterotubal ostia, known as "the tubal sunshine sign" **(Fig. 8)**. It is well known that tubal disease, and in particular hydrosalpinx, negatively impacts the outcome of IVF and that surgical management should be considered in all women with this diagnosis before undergoing ART.[52]

REFERENCES

1. Parry JP, Isaacson KB. Hysteroscopy and why macroscopic uterine factors matter for fertility? Fertil Steril. 2019;112(2):203-10.
2. Cicinelli E, Resta L, Nicoletti R, Tartagni M, Marinaccio M, Bulletti C, et al. Detection of chronic endometritis at fluid hysteroscopy. J Minim Invasive Gynecol. 2005;12(6):514-8.
3. Cicinelli E, De Ziegler D, Nicoletti R, Tinelli R, Saliani N, Resta L, et al. Poor reliability of vaginal and endocervical cultures for evaluating microbiology of endometrial cavity in women with chronic endometritis. Gynecol Obstet Invest. 2009;68(2):108-15.
4. Park HJ, Kim YS, Yoon TK, Lee WS. Chronic endometritis and infertility. Clin Exp Reprod Med. 2016;43(4):185-92.
5. Bosteels J, van Wessel S, Weyers S, Broekmans FJ, D'Hooghe TM, Bongers MY, et al. Hysteroscopy for treating subfertility associated with suspected major uterine cavity abnormalities. Cochrane Database Syst Rev. 2018;12(12): CD009461.
6. Volodarsky-Perel A, Badeghiesh A, Shrem G, Steiner N, Tulandi T. Chronic endometritis in fertile and infertile women who underwent hysteroscopic polypectomy. J Minim Invasive Gynecol. 2020;27(5):1112-8.
7. Salazar CA, Isaacson KB. Office Operative Hysteroscopy: An Update. J Minim Invasive Gynecol. 2018;25(2):199-208.
8. The Use of Hysteroscopy for the Diagnosis and Treatment of Intrauterine Pathology: ACOG Committee Opinion, Number 800. Obstet Gynecol. 2020; 135(3):e138-48.
9. Vitale SG, Ludwin A, Vilos GA, Török P, Tesarik J, Vitagliano A, et al. From hysteroscopy to laparoendoscopic surgery: what is the best surgical approach for symptomatic isthmocele? A systematic review and meta-analysis. Arch Gynecol Obstet. 2020;301(1):33-52.
10. López Rivero LP, Jaimes M, Camargo F, López-Bayghen E. Successful treatment with hysteroscopy for infertility due to isthmocele and hydrometra secondary to cesarean section: a case report. World J Clin Cases. 2019;7(6): 753-8.
11. Calzolari S, Sisti G, Pavone D, Ciocia E, Bianchini N, Cozzolino M. Prevalence of infertility among patients with isthmocele and fertility outcome after isthmocele surgical treatment: a retrospective study. Ochsner J. 2019 Fall;19(3):204-09.
12. Florio P, Filippeschi M, Moncini I, Marra E, Franchini M, Gubbini G. Hysteroscopic treatment of the cesarean-induced isthmocele in restoring infertility. Curr Opin Obstet Gynecol. 2012;24(3):180-6.
13. Sipahi S, Sasaki K, Miller CE. The minimally invasive approach to the symptomatic isthmocele: what does the literature say? A step-by-step primer on laparoscopic isthmocele—excision and repair. Curr Opin Obstet Gynecol. 2017;29(4):257-65.
14. Zhang J, Zou B, Wang K. Spontaneous expulsion of a huge cervical leiomyoma from the vagina after cesarean: A case report with literature review. Medicine (Baltimore). 2018;97(33):e11766.
15. Pakrashi T. New hysteroscopic techniques for submucosal uterine fibroids. Curr Opin Obstet Gynecol. 2014;26(4):308-13.

16. DI Spiezio Sardo A, Ceci O, Zizolfi B, Nappi C, Bettocchi S. Office myomectomy. Minerva Ginecol. 2016;68(3):321-7.
17. Veiga-Ferreira MM, Leiman G, Dunbar F, Margolius KA. Cervical endometriosis: Facilitated diagnosis by fine needle aspiration cytologic testing. Am J Obstet Gynecol. 1987;157:849-56.
18. Alonso Pacheco L, Laganà AS, Ghezzi F, Haimovich S, Azumendi Gómez P, Carugno J. Subtypes of T-shaped uterus. Fertil Steril. 2019 ;112(2):399-400.
19. Coelho Neto MA, Ludwin A, Petraglia F, Martins WP. Definition, prevalence, clinical relevance and treatment of T-shaped uterus: systematic review. Ultrasound Obstet Gynecol. 2021;57(3):366-77.
20. Uyar E, Usal D, Selam B, Cincik M, Bagis T. IVF outcomes after hysteroscopic metroplasty in patients with T-shaped uterus. Fertil Res Pract. 2019;5:15.
21. Grimbizis GF, Gordts S, Di Spiezio Sardo A, Brucker S, De Angelis C, Gergolet M, et al. The ESHRE/ESGE consensus on the classification of female genital tract congenital anomalies. Hum Reprod. 2013;28(8):2032-44.
22. Ludwin A, Lindheim SR. T-shaped uterus and subtle uterine variances: a need for reliable criteria. Fertil Steril. 2019;112(2):248-9.
23. Neal SA, Morin SJ, Werner MD, Gueye NA, Pirtea P, Scott RT Jr, et al. Three-dimensional ultrasound diagnosis of T-shaped uterus is associated with adverse pregnancy outcomes after embryo transfer. Reprod Biomed Online. 2019;39(5):777-83.
24. De Franciscis P, Riemma G, Schiattarella A, Cobellis L, Colacurci N, Vitale SG, et al. Impact of hysteroscopic metroplasty on reproductive outcomes of women with a dysmorphic uterus and recurrent miscarriages: a systematic review and meta-analysis. J Gynecol Obstet Hum Reprod. 2020;49(7):101763.
25. Garzon S, Laganà AS, Di Spiezio Sardo A, Alonso Pacheco L, Haimovich S, Carugno J, et al. Hysteroscopic metroplasty for T-shaped uterus: a systematic review and meta-analysis of reproductive outcomes. Obstet Gynecol Surv. 2020;75(7):431-44.
26. Chan YY, Jayaprakasan K, Tan A, Thornton JG, Coomarasamy A, Raine-Fenning NJ. Reproductive outcomes in women with congenital uterine anomalies: a systematic review. Ultrasound Obstet Gynecol. 2011;38(4):371-82.
27. Rikken JF, Kowalik CR, Emanuel MH, Mol BW, Van der Veen F, van Wely M, et al. Septum resection for women of reproductive age with a septate uterus. Cochrane Database Syst Rev. 2017;1(1):CD008576.
28. Shokeir TA, Shalan HM, El-Shafei MM. Significance of endometrial polyps detected hysteroscopically in eumenorrheic infertile women. J Obstet Gynaecol Res. 2004;30:84-9.
29. de Sá Rosa e de Silva ACJ, Rosa e Silva JC, Candido dos Reis FJ, Nogueira AA, Ferriani RA. Routine office hysteroscopy in the investigation of infertile couples before assisted reproduction. J Reprod Med. 2005;50:501-6.
30. Al Chami A, Saridogan E. Endometrial Polyps and Subfertility. J Obstet Gynaecol India. 2017;67(1):9-14.
31. Varasteh NN, Neuwirth RS, Levin B, Keltz MD. Pregnancy rates after hysteroscopic polypectomy and myomectomy in infertile women. Obstet Gynecol. 1999;94:168-71.
32. Perez-Medina T, Bajo-Arenas J, Salazar F, et al. Endometrial polyps and their implication in the pregnancy rates of patients undergoing intrauterine

insemination: a prospective, randomized study. Hum Reprod. 2005;20:1632-5. doi: 10.1093/humrep/deh822.

33. Nappi C, Di Spiezio Sardo A. Rare and difficult-to-interpret hysteroscopic findings. In: Nappi C, Di Spiezio Sardo A (Eds). State-of-the-art hysteroscopic approaches to pathologies of the genital tract. Tuttlingen: Endo-Press; 2014. pp. 236-49.
34. Puente E, Alonso L, Laganà AS, Ghezzi F, Casarin J, Carugno J. Chronic endometritis: old problem, novel insights and future challenges. Int J Fertil Steril. 2020;13(4):250-6. Published online 2019 Nov 11. doi: 10.22074/ijfs.2020.5779.
35. Song D, Li TC, Zhang Y, Feng X, Xia E, Huang X, et al. Correlation between hysteroscopy findings and chronic endometritis. Fertil Steril. 2019;111(4):772-9. doi: 10.1016/j.fertnstert.2018.12.007. Epub 2019 Jan 22.
36. Vitagliano A, Saccardi C, Noventa M, Di Spiezio Sardo A, Saccone G, Cicinelli E, et al. Effects of chronic endometritis therapy on in vitro fertilization outcome in women with repeated implantation failure: a systematic review and meta-analysis. Fertil Steril. 2018;110(1):103-12.e1. doi: 10.1016/j.fertnstert.2018.03.017. Epub 2018 Jun 13.
37. Lebovitz O, Orvieto R. Treating patients with "thin" endometrium—an ongoing challenge. Gynecol Endocrinol. 2014;30(6):409-14. doi: 10.3109/09513590.2014.906571. Epub 2014 Apr 2.
38. Garcia-Velasco JA, Acevedo B, Alvarez C, Alvarez M, Bellver J, Fontes J, et al. Strategies to manage refractory endometrium: state-of-the-art in 2016. Reprod Biomed Online. 2016;32(5):474-89. doi: 10.1016/j.rbmo.2016.02.001. Epub 2016 Feb 23.
39. Kasius A, Smit JG, Torrance HL, Eijkemans MJ, Mol BW, Opmeer BC, et al. Endometrial thickness and pregnancy rates after IVF: a systematic review and meta-analysis. Hum Reprod Update. 2014;20:530-41.
40. Munro MG. Uterine polyps, adenomyosis, leiomyomas, and endometrial receptivity. Fertil Steril. 2019;111(4):629-40. doi: 10.1016/j.fertnstert.2019.02.008.
41. Munro MG, Critchley HO, Broder MS, Fraser IS. FIGO Working Group on Menstrual Disorders. FIGO classification system (PALM-COEIN) for causes of abnormal uterine bleeding in nongravid women of reproductive age. Int J Gynaecol Obstet. 2011;113(1):3-13. doi: 10.1016/j.ijgo.2010.11.011. Epub 2011 Feb 22.
42. Capmas P, Voulgaropoulos A, Legendre G, Pourcelot AG, Fernandez H. Hysteroscopic resection of type 3 myoma: a new challenge? Eur J Obstet Gynecol Reprod Biol. 2016;205:165-9. doi: 10.1016/j.ejogrb.2016.06.026. Epub 2016 Aug 31.
43. Eldar-Geva T, Meagher S, Healy DL, MacLachlan V, Breheny S, Wood C. Effect of intramural, subserosal, and submucosal uterine fibroids on the outcome of assisted reproductive technology treatment. Fertil Steril. 1998;70:687-91.
44. Casini ML, Rossi F, Agostini R, Unfer V. Effects of the position of fibroids on fertility. Gynecol Endocrinol 2006;22:106-9.
45. Christopoulos G, Vlismas A, Salim R, Islam R, Trew G, Lavery S. Fibroids that do not distort the uterine cavity and IVF success rates: an observational study using extensive matching criteria. BJOG 2017;124:615-21.

46. Aghajanova L, Houshdaran S, Irwin JC, Giudice LC. Effects of noncavity-distorting fibroids on endometrial gene expression and function. Biol Reprod. 2017;97:564-76.
47. Yan L, Yu Q, Zhang YN, Guo Z, Li Z, Niu J, et al. Effect of type 3 intramural fibroids on in vitro fertilization-intracytoplasmic sperm injection outcomes: a retrospective cohort study. Fertil Steril 2018;109:817-22.e2.
48. Sunkara SK, Khairy M, El-Toukhy T, Khalaf Y, Coomarasamy A. The effect of intramural fibroids without uterine cavity involvement on the outcome of IVF treatment: a systematic review and meta-analysis. Hum Reprod. 2010;25: 418-29.
49. Metwally M, Farquhar CM, Li TC. Is another meta-analysis on the effects of intramural fibroids on reproductive outcomes needed? Reprod Biomed Online. 2011;23:2-14.
50. Chotaliya AB, Saifi SGA, Achuthan G. Sonographic appearance of endometrial osseous metaplasia. J Clin Ultrasound. 2018;46(8):536-9. doi: 10.1002/jcu.22587. Epub 2018 Mar 8.
51. Bettocchi S, Selvaggi L. A vaginoscopic approach to reduce the pain of office hysteroscopy. J Am Assoc Gynecol Laparosc. 1997;4(2):255-8.
52. Di Spiezio Sardo A, Bettocchi S, Bramante S, Greco E, Spinelli M, Nappi C. Tubal ostium sunshine: hysteroscopic sign of chronic salpingitis. J Minim Invasive Gynecol. 2012;19(6):676-7. doi: 10.1016/j.jmig.2012.01.011. PMID: 23084667.
53. Sedrati A, Drizi A, van Herendael B, Djokovic D. Hysteroscopic diagnosis of omentum incarceration subsequent to an iatrogenic uterine perforation. J Minim Invasive Gynecol. 2019;26(1):29-30. doi: 10.1016/j.jmig.2018.02.020. Epub 2018 Mar 7.
54. Moore JF, Carugno J. Hysteroscopy, 2020 Nov 20. In: StatPearls [Internet]. Treasure Island (FL): StatPearls Publishing; 2021 Jan. PMID: 33232015.
55. Vitale SG, Bruni S, Chiofalo B, Riemma G, Lasmar RB. Updates in office hysteroscopy: a practical decalogue to perform a correct procedure. Updates Surg. 2020;72(4):967-76. doi: 10.1007/s13304-020-00713-w. Epub 2020 Feb 1.
56. Vitale SG, Haimovich S, Riemma G, Ludwin A, Zizolfi B, De Angelis MC, Carugno J. Innovations in hysteroscopic surgery: expanding the meaning of "in-office". Minim Invasive Ther Allied Technol. 2020;23:1-8. doi: 10.1080/13645706.2020.1715437. Epub ahead of print.
57. Vitale SG, Carugno J, Riemma G, Török P, Cianci S, De Franciscis P, Parry JP. Hysteroscopy for assessing fallopian tubal obstruction: a systematic review and diagnostic test accuracy meta-analysis. J Minim Invasive Gynecol. 2021;28(4):769-78. doi: 10.1016/j.jmig.2020.11.013.

12

CHAPTER

Septum and Management Plan

Tanvir Singh

INTRODUCTION

Uterine septum represents 35% of congenital uterine malformations (CUM). It is the most common form.[1,2] Uterine septum has abnormal blood supply, increased muscle in the septum leading to uncoordinated uterine contractions, and decreased number of glandular and ciliated cells in the endomctrium. These factors increase the risk of infertility, implantation failure, recurrent miscarriage, and obstetrical complications.[3,4]

CLASSIFICATION AND TYPES

Two main classification systems are American Society for Reproductive Medicine and European Society of Human Reproduction and Embryology.

The ASRM American Fertility Society (AFS) classification, initially published in 1988, which was subsequently modified in 2016, 2021 and the European Society of Human Reproduction and Embryology (ESHRE)/ European Society for Gynaecological Endoscopy (ESGE) Working Group classification devised in 2014. **Table 1** expands on the details and comparison of both classifications.

The CONgenital UTerine Anomalies (CONUTA) ESHRE/European Society for Gynaecological Endoscopy Working Group, defined a septate uterus as a congenital uterine anomaly with pathological persistence of the median septum due to an abnormal resorption phenomenon, a normal outline of the uterine fundus.[5] This category is further divided into two subclasses (U2a and U2b), depending on whether the apex of the septum reaches the internal cervical os or stops above it **(Fig. 1)**.

PLANNING

In asymptomatic women, diagnosed septum, must be documented (ESGE). Should hysteroscopy metroplasty be performed?

This is one of the most controversial discussions. There are no randomized clinical trials to answer the question of whether metroplasty should be offered to patients with septum in primary infertility, especially prior to

TABLE 1: Features of ASRM and ESHRE—ESGE classification.

ASRM[6]	*ESHRE–ESGE*
2021	Working group—CONUTA (CONgenital UTerine Anomalies) devised the guidelines in 2016
Based on the American Fertility Society (AFS) classification. It is simple and reproducible	Based on the anatomy of female genital tract
It includes all categories of anomalies to improve clinical care	Anomalies are grouped based on clinical significance
Uses descriptive words, such as uterus didelphys, duplicated cervix, with obstructed right hemivagina and right renal agenesis	Uses terms such as U3 C2 V2 or VCUAM (V5a, C1, U2, A0, MR)
• Describes the various anomalies and the variations of the uterus, cervix and vagina. It has a more detailed diagrammatic representation of the variants of the anomalies • Provides user with surgical or medical options	Describes the various anomalies and the variations of the uterus, cervix and vagina
Gynecological examination should be performed	Gynecological examination should be performed
Ideal screening tool: Ultrasound or magnetic resonance imaging (MRI)	Diagnostic tool and accuracy in decreasing order: 3D-US (97.6%), sonohysterography (SHG: 96.5%), 2D US (86.6) and hysterosalpingography (HSG: 86.9%). MRI (90%)
Ideal diagnostic tool: MRI, during imaging, either by ultrasound or MRI, it is good to evaluate for aplastic or ectopic kidney	• 3D-US may be more accurate than MRI in sub-classifying malformations • Uterine wall thickness is the reference point to differentiate between dysmorphic T-shaped, septate and bicorporeal uteri
Ultrasound measurement in coronal plane with visible intramural parts of the tubal ostia *Septate uterus:* Fundal indentation of <1 cm and internal fundal indentation of >1.5 cm	Ultrasound measurement in sagittal plane at the thickest part. Uterine wall thickness is the reference point *Septate uterus:* Internal fundal indentations >50% of the uterine wall, and the depth of the external intercornual cleft was <50%
Possible risk of under diagnosis	Possible risk of over diagnosis of septate uterus

Source: For ASRM classification, *https://www.asrm.org/globalassets/_asrm/ practice-guidance/practice-guidelines/pdf mac2021_manuscript.pdf.*

in-vitro fertilization. The main indication for surgical removal of septum is poor obstetric outcome.

A systemic review and meta-analysis from 2022 found that uterine septum had a detrimental effect on pregnancy rate, live birth rate, spontaneous abortions and pregnancy loss. After septum removal: the proportion of live birth rate was higher (OR 49.58, 95% CI 29.93–82.13; p <0.0001) and the proportion of spontaneous abortion and pregnancy loss was lower after the removal of the septum (OR 0.02, 95% CI 0.02–0.04; p <0.000 and OR 0.05, 95% CI 0.03–0.08; p <0.0001).[3]

The European Society of Human Reproduction and Embryology (ESHRE), National Institute of Health and Care Excellence (NICE) and the Royal College of Obstetricians and Gynaecologists (RCOG) are not in favor of treating a septum for infertility.

TRUST (The Randomized Uterine Septum Trial) concluded the septum resection does not improve reproductive outcomes. Though this is a multicenter study including 10 centers, the limitations were the low sample size of 80, and the study lasted for a decade, and subgroup analysis of live birth rate, preterm birth, spontaneous abortion, recurrent pregnancy loss and infertility was not possible.[7, 8]

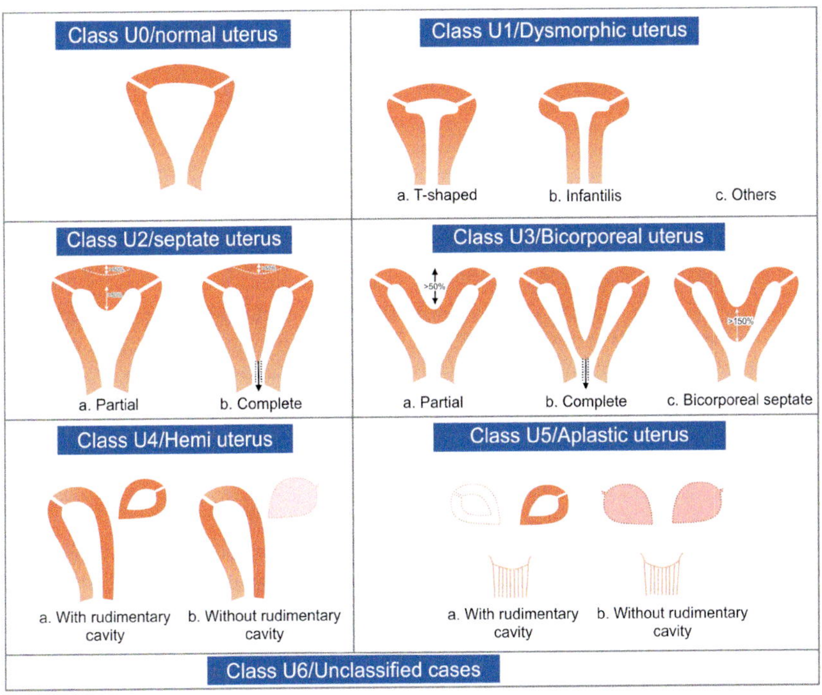

Fig. 1

Contd...

Contd...

ESHRE/ESGE classification
Female genital tract anomalies

	Uterine anomaly	
	Main class	***Sub-class***
U0	Normal uterus	
U1	Dysmorphic uterus	**a.** T-shaped **b.** Infantilis **c.** Others
U2	Sepate uterus	**a.** Partial **b.** Complete
U3		**a.** Partial **b.** Complete **c.** Bicroporal septate
U4	Hemi-uterus	**a.** With rudimentany cavity (communicating or not horn) b. Without rudimentary cavity (horn withtout cavity/no horn)
U5	Aplastic	**a.** With rudimentany cavity (bi- or unilateral horn) b. Without rudimentary cavity (bi- or unilateral uterine remnants/aplasia)
U6	**Unclassified malformation**	

Cervical/vaginal anomaly	
Co-existent class	
C0	*Normal cervix*
C1	*Septate cervix*
C2	*Double 'normal' cervix*
C3	*Unilateral cervical aplasia*
C4	*Cervical aplasia*
V0	*Normal vagina*
V1	*Longitudinal non-obstructing vaginal septum*
V2	*Longitudinal obstructing vaginal septum*
V3	*Transverse vaginal septum and/or imperforate hymen*
V4	*Vaginal aplasia*

U ***C*** ***V***

Associated anomalies of non-Müllerian origin:

Drawing of the anomaly

Fig. 1: ESHRE/ESGE classification of uterine anomalies: Schematic representation (Class U2: internal indentation 0.50% of the uterine wall thickness and external contour straight or with indentation, 50%, Class U3: external indentation. 50% of the uterine wall thickness, Class U3b: width of the fundal indentation at the midline. 150% of the uterine wall thickness).

OPERATIVE TIPS

Hysteroscopic metroplasty (HM) is preferably performed in the early proliferative phase. It can be performed in the operating theater or in office setting. Progesterone therapy can be administered prior to surgical correction to thin the endometrium.

Hysteroscopic, uterus is inspected starting from a panoramic view and visualizing both the ostia. Keeping both the tubal ostia under vision as a guiding point, a transverse incision is given in the midline of the septum.

This helps to avoid injury to the healthy myometrium. The fundal thickness is maintained at 10–15 mm.

The procedure is considered complete when both the ostia are visualized in a panoramic view with free side-to-side movement of the hysteroscope.

Uterine perforation usually occurs at the posterior wall, when the correct plane of incision is lost. Traditionally, prior to the advent of miniaturized instruments. HM was performed with 26-Fr or 22-Fr resectoscope using Collin's knife. These required cervical dilatation with Hegar's dilators. Now HM can be performed using 5-Fr instruments via 4 or 5 mm hysteroscope or 16-Fr mini-resectoscope in office or OR.

CONCLUSION

Follow-up ultrasound with a relook hysteroscopy can be performed to know the success of the procedure. Patients must always be counseled for a two-step procedure. We do know that treating septum improves reproductive and obstetric of both partial and complete septum. Though data is limited, hysteroscopic metroplasty should be offered to women with recurrent pregnancy loss, and infertility.

REFERENCES

1. Hollett-Caines J, Vilos GA, Abu-Rafea B, Ahmad R. Fertility and pregnancy outcomes following hysteroscopic septum division. J Obstet Gynaecol Can. 2006;28:156-9.
2. Grimbizis GF, Camus M, Tarlatzis BC, Bontis JN, Devroey P. Clinical implications of uterine malformations and hysteroscopic treatment results. Hum Reprod Update. 2001;7:161-74.
3. Noventa M, Spagnol G, Marchetti M, Saccardi C, Bonaldo G, Laganà AS, Cavallin F, Andrisani, A, Ambrosini G, Vitale SG, et al. Uterine septum with or without hysteroscopic metroplasty: impact on fertility and obstetrical outcomes—a systematic review and meta-analysis of observational research. J Clin Med. 2022;11:3290.
4. Chang Y, Shen M, Wang S, Guo Z, Duan H. Reproductive outcomes and risk factors of women with septate uterus after hysteroscopic metroplasty. Front Endocrinol. 2023;14:1063774.
5. Grimbizis GF, Di Spiezio Sardo A, et al. The Thessaloniki ESHRE/ESGE consensus on diagnosis of female genital anomalies. Gynecol Surg. 2016;13:1-16. doi: 10.1007/s10397-015-0909-1.
6. Pfeifer SM, Attaran M, Goldstein J, Lindheim SR, Petrozza JC, Rackow BW, et al. ASRM Müllerian anomalies classification 2021. Fertil Steril. 2021;116(5):1238-52. doi: 10.1016/j.fertnstert.2021.09.025. Erratum in: Fertil Steril. 2023;119(6):1088.
7. Rikken JFW, Kowalik CR, Emanuel MH, et al. Septum resection versus expectant management in women with a septate uterus: an international multicentre open-label randomized controlled trial. Hum Reprod. 2021;36(5):1260-7.
8. Ludwin A, Ludwin I. Comparison of the ESHRE-ESGE and ASRM classifications of Müllerian duct anomalies in everyday practice. Hum Reprod. 2015;30(3):569-80.

13 CHAPTER

Complications of Diagnostic and Surgical Hysteroscopy

Chaitanya Shembekar

Diagnostic and surgical hysteroscopic techniques have become established as primary techniques in gynecological practice and completely revolutionized the therapeutic approach in endocavitary pathology. Hysteroscopy is considered a minimally invasive procedure with low incidence of complications. Ozturk et al. report a complication rate of 0.86% in a retrospective study of 580 hysteroscopies, the most common being wrong ways and perforation.[1]

Endoscopic surgery complications are not only related to the surgeon's skill but also the use of operating instruments.

We can broadly divide complications as intraoperative and postoperative complications.

INTRAOPERATIVE COMPLICATIONS

- Pain and vasovagal crisis
- Trauma
- Hemorrhage
- Complications related to distension media
- Thermal damage caused by the electric current
- Infection

Pain and Vasovagal Crisis

Office hysteroscopy is becoming popular. Pain is an immediate complication where no form of anesthesia is used. The risk of vasovagal crisis is strictly related to pain. The pain is principally caused by excessive distension of the uterine cavity and by passage of instruments through the cervical canal. Some factors related to patients may favor the onset of symptoms such as chronic PID, nulliparity, menopause, anxiety. Invention of instruments increasingly reduced in diameter has noticeably reduced the incidence of such complications. Pain can be relieved by common analgesics, gentle hand movements while vasovagal syndrome is blocked with the use of atropine.[2]

Trauma

Most frequent trauma are uterine and cervical perforation, and laceration of the cervix. Documented cases in medical journals indicate that cervical and uterine perforations during hysteroscopy have variable incidence between 1–9%.[3] Cervical dilatation during resectoscope insertion are commonly associated with lacerations and perforations. Surgical techniques like metroplasty, myomectomy and endometrial resection or ablation carry a risk of uterine perforation. Pre-existing conditions like cervical stenosis, hyper-anteverted or hyper-retroverted uterus, atrophic post-menopausal uterus, uterine hypoplasia and endometrial carcinoma. Monitoring of such patients should be done using ultrasonography to exclude injury and bleeding and must be administered antibiotics and IV Oxytocin. Serious complications can be caused by a perforation induced by resectoscope electrode and require definitive management such as diagnostic laparoscopy or exploratory laparotomy to rule out injury to intra-abdominal organs like bladder, bowel and omentum.

A possible perforation is suspected in case of unexpected insufficient distension or hemorrhage and is diagnosed on the basis of direct hysteroscopic vision. The presence of abdominopelvic pain, fever, nausea, vomiting, leukocytosis and peritonitis following the procedure needs to be evaluated to diagnose the uterine perforation.[4]

Hemorrhage

Surgical corrective procedures such as submucous myomectomy or endometrial resection/ablation can cause uncontrolled bleeding. The expertise and ability of surgeon and use of incorrect instruments are also causative factors for bleeding. Intraoperatively a bleeder can be identified by reducing the pressure of distension media and minimal venous bleeding can be stopped by an increase in the pressure of distension media. Venous and arterial bleeding can be stopped using bipolar coagulation and/or IV administration of oxytocin to stimulate uterine contraction. The procedure must be suspended if the bleeding is uncontrolled and obscuring the operating field.

A Foley's catheter is inserted into the uterine cavity and uterine cavity is distended with 5 cc of normal saline and distension is gradually increased by 1 cc at a time if bleeding does not stop. Sudden distension is avoided to alleviate the risk of rupture. The cathcter must remain in the cavity for at-least 6 hours and ideally 24 hours. Hysterectomy is planned if the bleeding does not stop. In diagnostic hysteroscopy, vaginoscopy followed by entrance of into the cervical canal under vision reduces the risk of bleeding caused by tenaculum trauma or dilatation of cervical canal.[5]

Complications Related to Distension Media

Distension media for hysteroscopic surgery must be non-conducting if unipolar current is used. It is therefore important to use non-electrolytic low viscosity solutions for distension of uterine cavity (glycine, sorbitol-mannitol) to avoid propagating electric current with consequent thermal damage. Use of excessive quantity and rapid passage of distension media directly into the vessel causes fluid overload, electrolyte alteration and metabolic imbalance. The use of isotonic liquids like saline which can be used with bipolar current carries a risk of circulatory overload, serious damage to central nervous system, acute pulmonary edema, acute renal insufficiency or intravasation syndrome. The pathogenesis consists of an increase in central arterial and venous pressure in response to hypervolemia, which results in reduction in hematocrit and hyponatremia.[6] Symptoms are respiratory like dyspnea, pulmonary edema and neurological like headache, nausea, vomiting, agitation, convulsions. Signs include appearance of pale urine, tissue edema, increase in cardiac output with ventricular overload, variations of pulse oximetry and ventilatory parameters, variations in body temperature. Laboratory parameters show hypoproteinemia, hyponatremia and hemodilution. The causes which can provoke intravasation syndrome are the use of high intrauterine pressure (>80 mm Hg), duration of procedure and opening of consistent caliber myometrial vessels as in myomectomy, endometrial resection/ablation, metroplasty.

It is therefore fundamental to carefully monitor the duration of procedure (approx. 30 min) and quantity of distension fluid used. Use of electronically controlled irrigation and suction pump-like ENDOMAT is essential for constant control of intrauterine pressure, liquid flow, suction/irrigation pressure and the difference between quantity of fluid supplied and recovered. Kim et al. evaluated hyponatremia in patients who had undergone hysteroscopic surgery with resectoscope, and highlighted a greater risk in hysteroscopic myomectomy.[6] Episodes of gaseous embolism with liquid distension media has been described due to air contained in filling circuit which could accidentally penetrate wide uterine vessels. To prevent this, it is crucial to prime the irrigation circuit before the introduction of instrument.

CO_2 as a distension medium has been abandoned due to complications like CO_2 gas embolism and alterations in heart sounds described in literature.[7]

Now-a-days normal saline is used as a distension media and bipolar cautery is used for surgical procedures. This has drastically reduced the complications related to glycine as a distension media.

Prevention Methods for Fluid Overload Syndrome

- Locoregional anesthesia to keep patient awake
- Bipolar electric system with physiological solution for distension of uterine cavity
- Maintain distension pressures between 70–90 mm Hg
- Operate quickly to reduce surgery time
- Discrepancy volume should be less than 1.5 liters for saline, 1.5 liters for glycine and 1 liter for sorbitol, beyond which serum electrolytes must be evaluated.
- Collaboration with anesthetist
- Continuous communication with patients to identify any signs early such as cough, thoracic pressure or loss of consciousness.

Management of Intravasation Syndrome

- Immediately suspend the procedure at the onset of first symptom
- Use of IV Furosemide (20–40 mg)
- In case of specific symptomatology, increase natremia 1.5–2 mEq/L every 2 hours upto 135 mEq/L. Anti-shock treatment (3% hypertonic sodium chloride solution) containing 513 mEq/L and 3.33 times more osmotic than physiological solution.
- Avoid other IV fluids, if necessary only ringer lactate solution
- Laboratory examination every 2 hours like hemoglobin, hematocrit, proteins and Na^+, K^+ and Cl^- ions.

Diffusion of Neoplastic Tissue

This is prevented by the use of distension pressure <70 mm Hg, values corresponding to the opening pressure of tubal ostia.[8]

Thermal Damage Caused by Electric Current

With unipolar current, lesions can occur in different areas from the target due to electron flow following mistaken activation of the instrument, insulation problem with instrument and use of high power.

The use of bipolar current reduces this risk. To avoid thermal damage, it is advisable to activate the loop only under direct visual control and for brief periods. Modern HF electrosurgical units, specifically designed for endoscopic applications, should be used. These devices are electronically controlled and generate a variable intensity current depending on the tissue's resistance. The power is thus automatically regulated, so as to avoid possible complications from diffusion of unipolar current.

POSTOPERATIVE COMPLICATIONS

Postoperative complications are less common but more dangerous as it can occur in patients far away from hospital, as most of the hysteroscopy surgeries are daycare procedures.

Cases of postoperative hemorrhage have a low incidence.

Thermal damage to the bowel can go unnoticed during the procedure. The presence of abdominal pain, fever, leukocytosis can manifest after several days. Adequate medical therapy can reduce incidence.

Infections are rare complications. The incidence is 0.2–1% of all hysteroscopic procedures. Fever and abdominal pain manifest within 72 hours. This is prevented by skillful and rapid surgery, prophylactic antibiotics and correct sterilization of instruments.[9]

CONCLUSION

- Hysteroscopic surgery is considered a safe technique today.
- Complications are usually related to the skill and experience of surgeons.
- Training is crucial before attempting difficult procedures.
- Absolute requirement is the availability of appropriate instruments.

REFERENCES

1. Ozturk E, Ugur MG, Balat O, Kutlar I, Dikensoy E, Cebesoy B. An analysis of hysteroscopy experience over a seven-year period. Clin Exp Obstet Gynecol. 2010;37(2):150-1.
2. Cicinelli E. Hysteroscopy without anaesthesia: review of recent literature. J Minim Invasive Gynaecol. 2010;17(6):703-8.
3. Munro MG. Complications of hysteroscopic and uterine resectoscopic surgery. Obstet Gynecol Clin North Am. 2010;37(3):399-425. Review
4. Bradley LD. Complications in hysteroscopy: prevention, treatment and legal risk. Curr Opin Obstet Gynecol. 2002;14(4):409-15. Review
5. Cicinelli E. Diagnostic minihysteroscopy with vaginoscopic approach: rational and advantages. J Minim Invasive Gynecol. 2005;12:396-400.
6. Kim AH, Keltz MD, Arici A, Rosenberg M, Olive DL. Dilutional hyponatremia during hysteroscopic myomectomy with sorbitol-mannitol distension medium. J Am Assoc Gynecol Laparosc. 1995;2(2):237-42.
7. Litta P, Bonora M, Pozzan C, et al. Carbon dioxide versus normal saline in outpatient hysteroscopy. Hum Reprod. 2003;11:2446-9.
8. Polyzos NP, Mauri D, Tsioras S, Messini CI, Valachis A, Messini IS. Intraperitoneal dissemination of endometrial cancer cells after hysteroscopy: a systematic review and meta-analysis. Int J Gynecol Cancer. 2010;20(2):261-7. Review
9. Kasius JC, Broekmans FJ, Fauser BC, Devroey P, Fatemi HM. Antibiotic prophylaxis for hysteroscopy evaluation of uterine cavity. Fertil Steril. 2011;95(2):792-4. Epub 2010 Sep 24.